POWER BREATHING

Breathe Your Way to Inner Power, Stress Reduction, Performance Enhancement, Optimum Health & Fitness

Other Titles by the Author

Books
Vital Point Strikes
Ultimate Flexibility
Ultimate Fitness Through Martial Arts
Combat Strategy
The Art of Harmony
Teaching Martial Arts: The Way of The Master
Martial Arts Instructor's Desk Reference
1,001 Ways To Motivate Yourself & Others
Martial Arts After 40
Complete Taekwondo Poomsae
Taekwondo Kyorugi: Olympic Style Sparring
Muye Dobo Tongji: The Comprehensive Illustrated Manual of Martial
Arts of Ancient Korea

DVDs
Ultimate Flexibility
Power Breathing
Ultimate Fitness
Self-defense Encyclopedia
Jang Bong Patterns
Junsado: Combat Strategy
Junsado: Short Stick Combat (1 & 2)
Junsado: Long Stick
Junsado: Double Sticks
Wrist & Arresting Locks
Knife Defense (1 & 2)
Complete Kicking (1 & 2)
Complete Sparring (1 & 2)
Ultimate Kicking Drills
Aero Kicks
Top 100 Scoring Techniques
Taegeuk Poomsae
Palgwae Poomsae
and more

POWER BREATHING

BREATHE YOUR WAY TO INNER POWER, STRESS REDUCTION, PERFORMANCE ENHANCEMENT, OPTIMUM HEALTH & FITNESS

Sang H. Kim, Ph.D.

Turtle Press   Santa Fe

Photographer: Cynthia A. Kim

ISBN 978-1-934903-09-4
LCCN 2008036496

Printed in the United States of America

10 9 8 7 6 5 4 3 2 1 0

Warning-Disclaimer
This book is designed to provide information on specific skills used in martial arts and fitness training.
It is not the purpose of this book to reprint all the information that is otherwise available to the author,
publisher, printer or distributors, but instead to complement, amplify and supplement other texts. You
are urged to read all available material, learn as much as you wish about the subjects covered in this
book and tailor the information to your individual needs. Anyone practicing the skills presented in
this book should be physically capable to do so and have the permission of a licensed physician before
participating in this activity or any physical activity.

Every effort has been made to make this book as complete and accurate as possible. However, there
may be mistakes, both typographical and in content. Therefore, this text should be used only as a
general guide and not the ultimate source of information on the subjects presented here in this book
on any skill or subject. The purpose of this book is to provide information and entertain. The author,
publisher, printer and distributors shall neither have liability nor responsibility to any person or entity
with respect to loss or damages caused, or alleged to have been caused, directly or indirectly, by the
information contained in this book.

Library of Congress Cataloguing in Publication Data

Kim, Sang H.
  Power breathing / by Sang H. Kim. -- 1st ed.
    p. cm.
  ISBN 978-1-934903-09-4
  1. Martial arts--Training. 2. Breathing exercises. I. Title.
  GV1102.7.T7K55 2008
  613'.192--dc22
                          2008036496

The CIRCLES OF POWER BREATHING logo is
trademarked and copyrighted by Turtle Press Corporation.

Preface

Life begins from the first breath and ends with the last drop of breath. In between, we live. We were born to live long and Power Breathing is one way of promoting longevity and vitality. It will recharge your energy and help you perform better at work, at play and at rest.

Without being conscious of it, babies are masters of breathing, but somewhere along the way, we lose that naturalness. This book is a reminder of your original, innocent way of breathing. Although the techniques may appear a bit complicated at first, the goal is simply to recover your natural sense of breathing and, of course, to empower your inner self.

Mastery comes in all different forms. When a process is meaningful, the path of learning, discovering, and benefiting will set you free from being conscious of the road. To master Power Breathing, take the liberty to choose whatever subject or exercise you are interested in. That's the beginning. Then imitate. Through imitation, you'll find the method or technique that best fits your physical condition and skill level.

Be like a caterpillar: shed the layers of your old habits one at a time. Facing obstacles, be like water. Flow to the lowest level then fill up the space while building your foundation. In time, your strength will help you flow over your obstacles.

Happy Power Breathing!

Sang H. Kim
Atalaya Mountain, summer 2008

Dedication

To Cynthia and Jessica and Dixie and Emma.

Acknowledgements

Many thanks to my teachers in martial arts training for the past four decades, particularly to Grandmaster Park Yong-tak and Grandmaster Kim Do-bu. Learning seems to be the passage toward enlightenment of not knowing. It took only decades to appreciate what had been taught and render validity to my doubt. I also thank my students for their support and dedication.

Notes to the Readers

Personal well-being is a high priority for many people: to be free of disease, to be free of fear, to have a sense of inner strength and physical capacity. Power Breathing is geared to reducing the factors that obstruct our well-being and enhancing those that contribute to well-being. As you practice the exercises and techniques in this book, keep in mind that a sensible approach and gradual, persistent progression are the keys to success. Should you have any medical concerns, consult your doctor before engaging in this program. If you feel dizziness or discomfort during an exercise, stop immediately and consult with a medical professional.

Contents

How to Use the Book

You may read this book from the beginning to the end, or flip to any page and practice a technique or exercise that interests you. If you are new to Power Breathing exercises or to breathing exercises in general, begin with the basic exercises in Chapter 3 then progress to Gentle Breathing and finally to the more strenuous Power Breathing methods. To get a better understanding of Power Breathing in action, you may also find it helpful to watch the *Power Breathing for Life DVD*, which includes several Power Breathing workouts using the exercises in this book as well as detailed instruction on the five Power Breathing methods.

As you become familiar with the methods taught here, you can incorporate Power Breathing techniques into literally any activity that you do in daily life - walking, running, playing tennis, gardening, riding the bus - anything! As you progress, you'll find that you are adapting Power Breathing techniques in ways that suit your body and your lifestyle.

FOR YOUR SAFETY: Power Breathing is a strenuous exercise. You should progressively increase the intensity and duration of practice for your safety. If you have a pulmonary, cardiac or auditory illness or any condition that might be adversely affected by the exercises presented in this book, consult your doctor before engaging in Power Breathing practice.

Holding your breath during condensing requires caution. Begin from your most comfortable level and gradually increase the length and intensity of condensing, conservatively adding one second at a time as you improve your capacity. Although we think of breathing as a natural daily activity, altering your breathing can be as stressful to the body as strenuous exercise and should be approached with the caution and common sense that you would approach any physically strenuous activity.

老子道德經第十章：

專氣致柔，
能嬰兒乎？

"When you pay undivided attention to your vital breathing, won't the body becomes as supple as a newborn baby?"
(Chapter 10, Tao Te Ching)

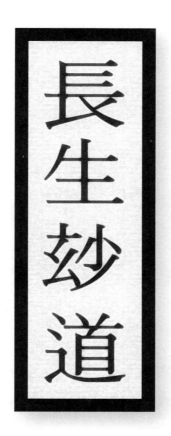

長生玅道: *an amazing way to longevity*

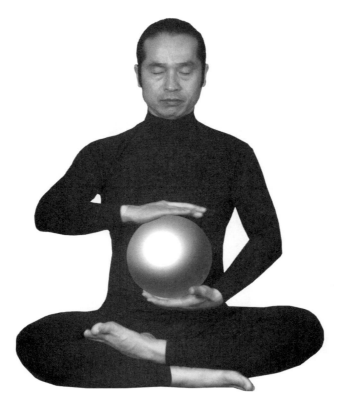

" Without knowing it,
once we were breathing masters. "

1

INTRODUCTION

A NEW LOOK AT BREATHING

Breathing is everything and everything else is in-between. It is the first thing we did at birth and the last thing we do when life expires. Living means breathing and breathing means living. One breath reaches a quadrillion cells, over 600 muscles, 62,000 miles of blood vessels and 300 million air sacs in the lungs.

For thousands of years, ancient masters and gurus of various forms of fitness have pursued the art of breathing to enhance their health and prolong their life span. Power Breathing is a method of breathing that can enhance your well-being, reduce your stress levels, improve your athletic performance, sharpen your concentration and increase your inner power.

Power Breathing not only strengthens your inner force but also enlarges the inner space in your torso to encourage optimal function of your organs. Insufficient room for breathing means an insufficient supply of oxygen, and a shortage of oxygen limits energy production in the cells. So facilitating enough room for the intake of oxygen is the first step in Power Breathing and the first step toward increasing your inner power. Once you have learned to increase your oxygen intake, you can strengthen your internal muscles and learn to harness your natural inner power.

How does it work? Power Breathing makes active changes in the way we breathe. By consciously modifying your method of breathing, you can optimize your bodily functions at the unconscious level. When your unconscious being is in balance, you will feel strong and energized at the conscious level. But how? The secret is to expand your inner space, to strengthen your inner muscles, to infuse sufficient oxygen into your blood stream and to cleanse the toxins from your body. These processes are accomplished by beginning with one simple change of habit: moving from lung breathing to belly breathing. Once you master belly breathing, Power Breathing takes the process one step further than most breathing methods by adding a condensing stage during which you intensely focus all of the body's energy in a single point while tensing your muscles and holding the breath.

BREATHING AND POWER

Power Breathing converts the mechanical work of the diaphragm and the belly muscles into vital energy. By elevating the pressure in the cavities of the torso and forcing the entire body to expand and contract along with the expansion and contraction of the diaphragm muscle, you increase the "horsepower" of your body. As the power and depth of your inhalation and exhalation increases, the vital organs in your torso are "massaged" by the movement of your diaphragm and belly muscles, enhancing the health and function of the organs. As you take in more oxygen, your muscles become "well fed" and able to work longer and harder. Your circulation will increase and the secretion of hormones will in turn be boosted, lubricating all of the body's key systems and delivering oxygen rich blood to the brain and spinal cord, the muscles and organs and to all of the cells of the body.

Deep, focused breathing sets off a series of chain reactions that keep the body functioning optimally. In turn, your performance - whether your athletic performance or your ability to take on your day with vigor - becomes more powerful and dynamic. You can generate more power using less of your vital energy and your ability to focus your inner power will be significantly increased.

Power Breathing can:

- Improve stamina
- Enhance muscular power
- Improve the mind-body connection
- Increase concentration
- Allow you to work longer and harder

- Decrease stress
- Reduce susceptibility to disease
- Strengthen the pelvic muscles
- Improve posture and attitude
- Enhance overall well-being

POWER BREATHING IN ACTION

Before we look at the methods and techniques of Power Breathing, let's look at how it might benefit you in your daily life.

Power Breathing at Play

Whether you are serious about your fitness, a "weekend warrior" or just getting started on a fitness plan, applying the methods of Power Breathing to your fitness routine can help you play harder and smarter. Power Breathing not only increases your lung capacity, leading to greater endurance, but it helps your body use the oxygen it takes in more efficiently. You'll find that your mind-body connection increases as you become conscious of the way your breath interacts with your movement.

Power Breathing at Work

Think breathing is just for exercise? Think again. Deep breathing increases the oxygen in your blood and well oxygenated blood in the brain is essential to clear thinking. If you feel your concentration waning during the day, a short session of Power Breathing in your office can refresh your thinking and allow you to return to work with renewed focus.

Power Breathing at Rest

Stress is one of the most frequent complaints that the average adult has about his or her health. Spending even five minutes a day for Power Breathing can markedly reduce your stress and leave you feeling energetic and positive rather than tired and distracted. Power Breathing brings your focus to one point, your breath, allowing you to let go of distracting thoughts while engaging in a moderately strenuous full body stretch. Because Power Breathing uses active, dynamic movements to open the chest and expand the belly, it reduces tension in areas where it tends to accumulate most - the upper torso, back, shoulders and neck.

Power Breathing as Healing

Many ailments that plague us today are vague and hard to cure - back pain, neck pain, joint pain, insomnia, tension, and anxiety are frequent complaints as we grow older. But many of these can be lessened or even banished from our lives through deep breathing and mindful movements. Power Breathing addresses these symptoms through the use of Gentle and Healing Breathing exercises that aim to stretch and strengthen the body while focusing on the breath, a time honored way of bringing the body back to health that has been used in Eastern cultures for centuries.

WHAT IS POWER BREATHING?

Power breathing is a controlled dynamic method of inhaling, condensing and then exhaling through movement to build inner strength. It can be done while sitting or lying down, but it is most potent when performed dynamically, while standing or moving. Power Breathing engages the whole body, internally and externally, by synchronizing deep breathing with complementary movements of the arms, legs and torso to bring the mind and body into oneness.

The postures and movements of Power Breathing balance and counterbalance the body's energy flow and stimulate specific parts of the body. Detailed explanations of the exercises and their benefits are in Chapters 3 through 8.

Small Things First

Mastery of a new activity can be overwhelming. You might feel that it takes too much time and there are too many rules to follow to understand everything. But take heart - you don't need to learn everything at once. Here are some key concepts to help you get started:

The Belly: Energy Hub

In breathing, we take in oxygen through the nose or mouth to fill the lungs, which are the hub for oxygen distribution. In Power Breathing, there is a second hub in the lower belly, which becomes the center of energy distribution. The belly muscles enhance the depth of breathing by creating space into which the lungs and diaphragm can descend, allowing a greater intake of air. If you look at the location of your lungs in your chest and the location of your belly, you can see why belly breathing requires that you breathe twice as deeply as lung breathing.

Longer Breathing for Longevity

There is a saying, "Short breath, short life. Long breath, long life." Although this sounds good, it is not always easy for beginners to suddenly breathe twice as deeply. So begin from the way you normally breathe and gradually extend the length. If one breath (one inhalation and exhalation) takes three seconds, try to make it four seconds. When you get comfortable with four seconds, try five seconds.

Natural Expansion

If you continue lung breathing, you'll find a limit in extending the length of your breath. Lung breathing is shallow and short; belly breathing is deep and long. Belly breathing is also more natural and holistic, making it easier to prolong. Whereas lung breathing forces the diaphragm to move down (inhaling) and up (exhaling), belly breathing creates a big space between the belly and lungs, into which the diaphragm is naturally lowered; when the belly is fully extended, the diaphragm leads the way in exhaling, moving upward, and forcing toxic air out while the belly naturally contracts. Additionally, moving the belly in and out stimulates your organs, almost like an internal massage, which boosts blood circulation in the stomach and visceral organs. The belly is the control center, initiating inhalation then following the natural process of exhalation; it is the core for Power Breathing.

The Magic Stone

Although the belly is the core of Power Breathing, it needs our imagination to give it life. The exact point of the center of the belly is abstract and imaginary, but this is where you need to visualize putting things together in order to make sense of what is happening in your body. The belly becomes meaningful in breathing through an abstract life force, when your conscious visualization accompanies the physical process of expanding the belly.

For centuries, it has been believed that there is a secret energy field hidden in the center of the belly - an invisible round ball of energy, known as the magic stone. It is also believed that life energy (known as Ki, Qi, Chi, or Prana) circulates throughout the body, nourishing and healing it. This healing energy is accumulative and is stored in the magic stone, connecting the body to the cosmic energy of the universe.

The Unconscious Consciousness

When you were a baby, belly breathing was natural for you, but now it requires conscious effort. Your habit, as an adult, is lung breathing. To change a habit, it takes 21 days of conscious effort. Until you establish the habit of Power Breathing, you need to consciously intervene in what your body is doing and be mindful of how your actions affect your body. With each day's successful practice, your body will gradually learn to take care of itself without your conscious intervention. Then, Power Breathing becomes your natural breathing for life.

" Emptiness is useful for fullness:
They are yin and yang of oneness."

2

POWER BREATHING PRINCIPLES

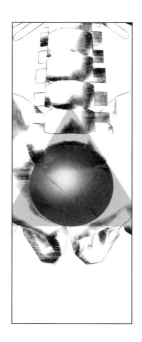

When you expand your lungs, air from outside rushes in to fill the void. This is a natural phenomenon of stabilizing an imbalance of pressure in the chest cavity.

In Power Breathing, you deliberately create this phenomenon by expanding the muscles of the lower abdomen. When you expand your lower abdomen, the diaphragm automatically moves downward creating more space for your lungs and this expansion pulls air into your lungs. When your lungs are filled, hold your breath for a moment and condense it downward. Once your lower abdomen is fully expanded, it naturally bounces back. All you need to do is slowly let it go (Gentle Breathing); tighten the muscles and intensify the force (Power Breathing); or move mindfully according to the position of your diaphragm (Healing Breathing).

The more air you pull in, the more power you can generate. The harder you condense the air, the more forceful the release is; thus it is called Power Breathing.

BREATHING METHODS COMPARISON

Lung Breathing

What happens:

As you inhale during lung breathing, the lungs enlarge and the belly is tucked in. A flat belly looks good but what happens inside the body is not a good thing. Instead of making the thoracic (chest) cavity larger vertically so that the lungs expand downward, the lungs are forced to expand forward. (The lungs cannot expand to the rear, toward the spine, or upward toward the clavicle.) In lung breathing the lungs and the diaphragm are forced to move unnaturally, resulting in shallow breathing.

Problems:

1) The lungs are forced to expand forward instead of downward.
2) The diaphragm is constricted and has nowhere to go to.
3) Breathing becomes short and shallow.
4) Less than maximum intake of oxygen into the blood stream.

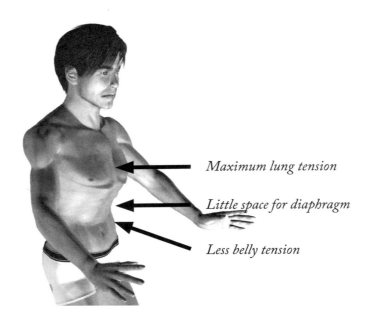

Maximum lung tension

Little space for diaphragm

Less belly tension

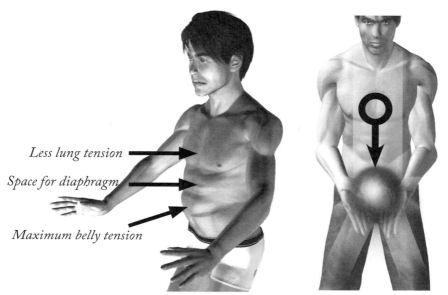

Less lung tension

Space for diaphragm

Maximum belly tension

The diaphragm (left) and condensing (right) in Power Breathing.

Diaphragm Breathing

What happens:

As you expand the lower belly, the abdominopelvic cavity becomes larger and the diaphragm naturally drops, creating space in the thoracic (chest) cavity which allows the lungs to expand downward. Air then enters through the nostrils and trachea, into the lungs in the enlarged thoracic vacuum. In diaphragm breathing, the diaphragm descends downward further than in lung breathing, bringing more oxygen into the body.

Power Breathing

What happens:

In Power Breathing, you take diaphragm breathing one step further. At completion of inhalation, when the belly muscles expand and the diaphragm descends, you hold the breath momentarily and tense all of the core muscles. Imagine a ball of energy forming and with active visualization, hold the ball and compress it downward by tensing your inner muscles. This is called the condensing stage, a breathing stage unique to Power Breathing.

POWER BREATHING: HOW IT WORKS

Power Breathing is an organic dynamic purposeful breathing method to generate optimal inner force for maximum circulation in the body. The goals of Power Breathing are to supply abundant oxygen to the cells and remove toxins from the body while strengthening the core muscles and increasing breathing capacity.

Broadly speaking, Power Breathing is a forced gas exchange between two spaces: the external environment and the body. The exchange takes place by diffusion: air moves in from a high concentration space to a lower concentration space. As this happens, our body uptakes fresh oxygen through inhalation and discharges toxic wastes through exhalation. This facilitates a constant circulation and renewal of life energy. Once the oxygen enters the body, it enters into the bloodstream and travels to the cells riding in hemoglobin. Power Breathing plays two significant roles in this process. One, by condensing, Power Breathing increases the inner force which accelerates circulation. Two, through regulation of the exhalation speed, Power Breathing holds air in the lungs longer, allowing the body to absorb more oxygen.

Physiologically, Power Breathing is a holistic strengthening exercise for the inner muscles and organs. It maximizes blood and oxygen flow, raises the body temperature, and restores inner power. Physically, Power Breathing is a transformation of infinite ambient air into a finite controllable energy form to increase the vitality in the body.

THREE STEPS OF POWER BREATHING

Normal breathing has two steps: inhalation and exhalation. Power Breathing has an additional step called condensing. The basic principle of Power Breathing is: inhaling—condensing—exhaling. However, there are many variations on this basic concept and you will see that many of the exercises break up the basic exhaling into a forceful exhalation and a more gentle releasing phase, separated by one or more condensing phases.

As ambient air enters the body, it converges in the lungs. When you suspend your breath momentarily at this point, you can create and hold a balloon-like bag of air in the torso. By contracting the inner muscles in the belly and mobilizing your active imagination, you can then press it downward to build pressure under the diaphragm. This condensing process is, in fact, an isometric inner muscle strengthening exercise. By suspending the breath and tensing the entire body, you can focus a great amount of force around a single point.

Inhalation

When the diaphragm descends during inhalation, the pressure in the thoracic cavity becomes lower than the environment and ambient air fluxes into the body. The diaphragm functions like a suction cup and air fills the lungs. The oxygen in the air is then transferred to the bloodstream as the blood flows by the lungs. The more air you are able to inhale, the more oxygen that will be available to the passing blood and in turn to the rest of the body.

Condensing

When air enters the lungs, the pressure in the thoracic cavity increases. If you exhale immediately, this is normal breathing and a normal amount of oxygen will be taken into the bloodstream. Power Breathing intensifies the breath by increasing the pressure in the thoracic cavity and then transferring that increased pressure to the center of the body through the process of condensing.

The diaphragm divides the torso into two areas: the thoracic and abdominopelvic cavities. When the lungs become full of oxygen during inhalation, the pressure in the thoracic cavity increases, which has excellent potential energy for internally strengthening the body. In Power Breathing, the intensity of the breath transfers the thoracic pressure down to the abdominal cavity by tensing the muscles in the belly and chest and the pelvic diaphragm and by using your active imagination.

During the condensing stage, you can drive the energy of the inhaled breath down through the diaphragm by forming an imaginary ball called the Golden Ball, located between the abdominal and pelvic cavities. This process generates highly concentrated and condensed energy that can increase circulation, raise the body temperature and generate vital life force.

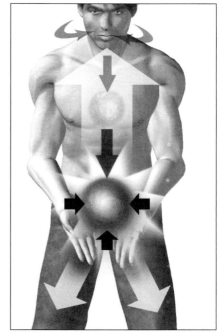

Grey arrow: Inhalation
Black arrow: Condensing
White arrows: Energy distribution
Upper circle: Holding the breath
Lower circle: Golden Ball

The duration for condensing is limited to a matter of seconds since it should be performed before the pressure is relieved by exhalation. Basically condensing is an interim process between inhalation and exhalation that builds internal force and intensifies the breath.

Because the pressure in the abdominopelvic cavity during Power Breathing rises higher than during normal breathing, condensing must be controlled by the intensity of the contraction of the belly muscles. Begin with gentle condensing to prepare your inner muscles and avoid straining. Power Breathing should not be work. You should be able to enjoy it and get the benefits of it, both immediately and in the long run.

Ultimately, condensing will improve the efficiency of energy distribution in the body by overcoming the limitations of regular breathing.

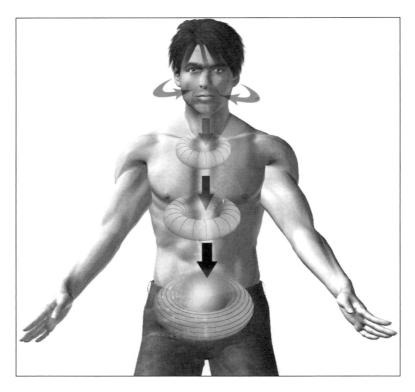

During condensing, imagine your energy traveling downward to your lower abdomen and forming a hard Golden Ball.

The Point of Condensing

Condensing primarily involves the diaphragm, the muscles in the belly and pelvic floor with assistance from the intercostal muscles. When you have mastered condensing, here is the process that occurs:

1. As the diaphragm hits the lowest point (at maximum contraction), the pelvic diaphragm (at the base of the pelvis) and belly muscles contract simultaneously.

2. The diaphragm pauses creating downward pressure, the pelvic diaphragm pushes the imaginary Golden Ball upward and the belly muscles press the Golden Ball against the spine.

3. The Golden Ball is condensed in the abdominal and pelvic cavities. The inner pressure in the body reaches maximum at this point. It requires concentration and active visualization to control the timing and position of the Golden Ball. Condensing usually lasts for 3 to 8 seconds. This is the only time when the diaphragm, the muscles of the belly and pelvic floor contract at the same time.

* Keep in mind that the Golden Ball is an imaginary tool that you can use to visualize the movement of energy in your body. It is formed by tensing your diaphragm, belly and pelvic muscles simultaneously. Achieving the condensing sequence can take a great deal of practice. You can master it by regularly practicing controlling, contracting and releasing your internal muscles. More detailed instruction on condensing is included with the descriptions of many of the exercises in Chapters 4 through 8.

Exhalation

In Power Breathing, exhalation is when the condensed energy is released unhurriedly. In fact, the more slowly you exhale, the better. During exhalation, focus on controlling the speed of the ascending diaphragm and contraction of the belly muscles and the pelvic diaphragm.

In some Power Breathing exercises, the exhalation is broken up, with part of it occurring before the condensing stage (called exhalation) and part of it occurring after condensing (called release). A detailed explanation of the order of the stages is included with each exercise and once you begin to understand the relationship of condensing and exhaling, you can experiment further on your own.

THREE STEPS OF POWER BREATHING - SUMMARY

There are three steps in Power Breathing: inhalation, condensing, and exhalation. Inhalation is the action of letting fresh air into the lungs and exhalation is the action of expelling carbon dioxide and other wastes from the body. Exhalation takes twice as long (or longer) as inhalation.

Inhalation:

A good analogy of inhalation is a bull pulling a man. The forceful belly muscles expand and pull the maximum amount of ambient air into the lungs. For hygiene, it is better to breathe in through the nose than the mouth. Nose inhalation cleans, humidifies and warms the air before it enters the lungs.

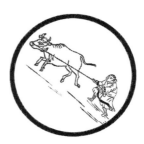

Condensing:

At this point, all of the muscles in the body contract, energy is forced toward a single point (the Golden Ball) and the pressure in the body reaches the maximum.

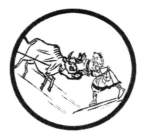

Exhalation:

This is when oxygen is transferred to the bloodstream and transported to the cells and toxins are collected for expulsion from the body. Drag the process as long as possible like restraining a lunging bull. You may exhale by either the nose or mouth, however mouth exhalation allows better control of the volume of exhalation.

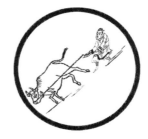

POWER BREATHING KEYS

There are three key elements emphasized in Power Breathing: posture, space, and control.

Forming Good Posture

Good posture is essential to good health. Posture is like a house: a well-built house provides room for safe and healthy living for the resident; a faulty structure impedes living activities and causes unsafe conditions. Similarly, improper posture induces stress and discomfort in the back, shoulders and neck and hinders the normal function of the organs and muscles. The fragile cavities of the torso, especially the abdominal cavity, become weaker when they are not well supported and protected by the framework of the skeleton.

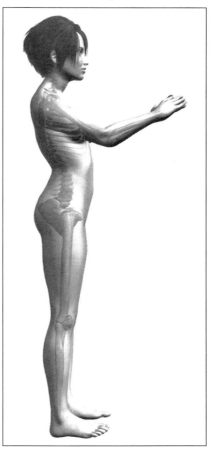

Good posture, however, enables your body to work naturally, in a strong and balanced manner with minimal stress to the spine, joints, and muscles. A properly aligned body optimizes the balance and proportion of the body structure. So what is good posture? Ideally, the spine has three natural curves: a slight forward curve in the lumbar (low back) region, a slight backward curve in the

ANCHOR THE BODY

There are four areas of the posture to anchor in Power Breathing to generate maximum power.

· Plant your feet firmly to anchor your base.
· Rest your pelvis on your lower limbs.
· Align your torso to create optimal space for the lungs and heart.
· Hold your head straight and fix your eyes to stabilize your balance.

thoracic (chest) region, and a slight extension in the top cervical (neck) vertebra. When the spine is properly aligned and erect, there is ample space in the torso for optimal breathing and circulation, as well as proper placement and functioning of the internal organs.

Restoring Space for Breathing

Space is important to relaxation and productivity. It is hard to relax in a cramped room or to produce things in crowded environment. Similarly, the organs in the body need space to contract and relax, to produce blood and hormones, and to digest and distribute nutrients. Power Breathing maximizes the inner space of the torso and stimulates the organs and nerves in the major cavities of the body through condensing and intensifying the inner pressure and increasing circulation.

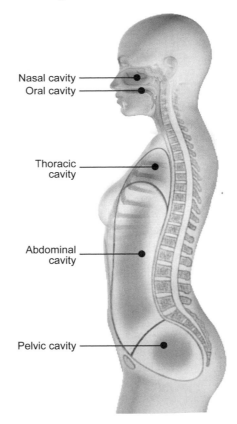

Nasal cavity

Oral cavity

Thoracic cavity

Abdominal cavity

Pelvic cavity

Control

Control, in Power Breathing, is the regulation of tension in your muscles either by extension or contraction, to limit or extend the length of each inhalation, condensing or exhalation. By intensely contracting your inner muscles, you can produce maximum force in the cavities of the torso. By deliberately slowing the ascending diaphragm, you can extend your exhalation and provide a larger volume of oxygen over a prolonged period to your body. With good control, you can adjust the volume, intensity and speed of energy being used in the same way you would turn the thermostat up or down according to how much heat you need to warm your house.

BREATHING POWER COMES FROM...

Condensing Power

Condensing power harnesses the strength of your inner muscles. The more capacity your inner muscles have to withstand the forces of the compressed air, the more condensing power you can generate. Imagine that you are pushing a car: first you put your hands on the rear of the car, move your feet back and bend your knees, then you inhale and push. In this scenario, the condensing stage occurs just before you begin to push the car. You've set your body, tensed your muscles, taken a deep breath and recruited all of your muscles to move the car. The more resistance there is, the more condensing power you need to generate to move the vehicle. The car will not move when your force is smaller than the resisting force of the car.

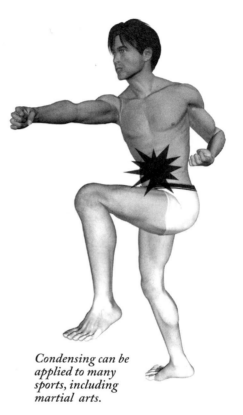

Condensing can be applied to many sports, including martial arts.

For more power, breathe deeply, lowering the diaphragm as far as you can to create more inner tension. Once you've inhaled fully and condensed the air, exhale slowly with control so you don't lose the power you've created. Remember the car example? Once the car begins to move, you'll begin exhaling slowly with absolute control so that you can continue pushing the car with power. If you just let your breath out as soon as you begin to move the car, your body will relax and you'll lose your momentum. This is a practical example of how Power Breathing is applied to a strenuous physical activity to generate added power and focus.

Hopefully now the concept of condensing makes sense in a more practical way. Condensing is a way to recruit a sudden burst of energy and apply it to the physical task at hand or to refresh your mental state by delivering a burst of oxygen to the brain. Once you understand the principles of Power Breathing, you can directly apply them to many activities including your favorite sport.

Diaphragm Tension

Because the diaphragm is a muscle, it is elastic and resilient. When you contract the diaphragm during inhalation, you create tension, much like drawing back a bow. Once the bow is drawn, you have to work hard to maintain the drawn position. Similarly, once the diaphragm is drawn downward, you have to consciously work to keep it from immediately returning to the naturally relaxed position.

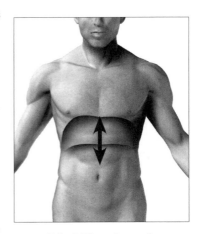

Much like a drawn bow, the diaphragm creates tension.

In Power Breathing, you should let the diaphragm return to its original position as slowly as possible by controlling the abdominal muscles. Imagine that you have pulled the string of the bow back and are slowly returning it to the original position using the resisting power of your arm muscles rather than letting it snap back. In Power Breathing, your belly muscles function like your arm muscles restraining the bow.

TENSION: SOURCE OF POWER

Tension is a source of strength. Your muscles create tension against each other and you can apply tension externally against your muscles, in the form of a weight or resistance. Just like building your muscles using weights, the amount of tension in Power Breathing determines the amount of inner force you can generate. When you lift a heavy weight, you create a great deal of tension in your muscles, forcing them to work hard and grow larger. In breathing, when you draw the diaphragm deeply downward and apply resistance as it returns to its normal state, you create inner tension, which strengthens the diaphragm and increases your inner power.

WHY POWER BREATHING?

The great Taoist sage Chuang Tzu says that most men breathe from the throats, but the wise breathe from their heels. Breathing enables us to reach the deepest realm of our self because our consciousness depends upon breath.

Deep and powerful breathing affects our conscious actions which not only changes our appearance into a more relaxed and self-confident one, but also changes our unconscious behavior into a more energetic and positive attitude. This is why many people feel a deep and lasting change in their physical and mental condition after beginning a regular program of Power Breathing.

Power Breathing is a purposeful mind-body training method: each breath slows the speed of the mind to bring it in sync with that of the body, gradually fading out the borders between them. Even after a short practice session, conscious thought significantly decreases and unconscious awareness increases. Our true power comes from that not-yet-known self and Power Breathing connects us to that link.

Most of us spend lots of time worrying about or suffering from some kind of pain or ailment. We are free yet we are not. But when our body becomes full of energy and power, in the absence of pain, disease and worries, we can fully function as a living being doing what we enjoy.

Power Breathing enables you to be energetic, awake, responsive and confident. Your mind will be fully related to your body without separation allowing you to be yourself again. Power Breathing makes free use of oxygen and natural law. The only price you need to pay is your action and imagination. It's up to you to take hold of the gift.

BREATHING PHYSIOLOGY

Before moving on to the exercises, you may find it helpful to understand what muscles you'll be engaging in Power Breathing, how those muscles affect the breath and how oxygen travels through the body. While this information isn't necessarily essential to being able to do the exercises correctly, understanding the anatomical basis for the exercises can assist you in visualizing which muscles are working and how.

Muscles for Inhalation

Contracting: diaphragm, external intercostal muscles
Expanding: rectus abdominis, transversus abdominis

Muscles for Condensing

Tensing: diaphragm, transversus abdominis, rectus abdominis, intercostal muscles, pelvic diaphragm

Muscles for Exhalation

Contracting: rectus abdominis, transversus abdominis, internal intercostal muscles, pelvic diaphragm
Relaxing: diaphragm

Core Muscles

Diaphragm

The thoracic diaphragm is the primary muscle in breathing. There are two thoracic diaphragms: a Crural (smaller) and a Costal (larger) diaphragm. In most cases, we use the crural diaphragm which is an involuntary muscle over which we have little or no control. The costal diaphragm, which controls the movement of the rib cage, is a voluntary muscle that we can control. During inhalation, the ribs expand and the diaphragm contracts and descends creating a vacuum in the thoracic (chest) cavity and drawing air into the lungs. During exhalation, the ribs contract and the diaphragm relaxes.

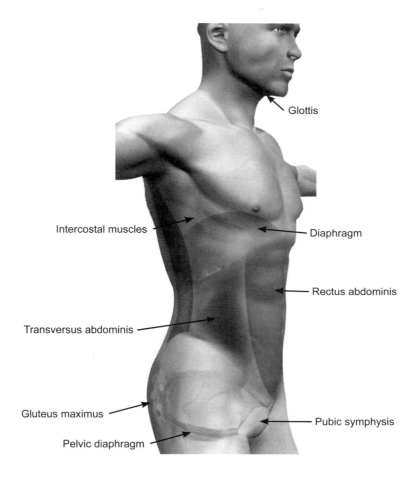

Glottis

Intercostal muscles

Diaphragm

Rectus abdominis

Transversus abdominis

Gluteus maximus

Pubic symphysis

Pelvic diaphragm

Intercostal Muscles

The intercostal muscles are three layers of muscles that run between the ribs, forming and mobilizing the chest wall. They are the prime movers in chest breathing. The external intercostal muscles assist in inhalation, lifting the ribs and expanding the chest cavity. The internal intercostal muscles assist in forced exhalation, as in Power Breathing, by depressing the rib cage and contracting the chest cavity. The innermost intercostal muscles, subcostal muscles and transversus thoracic muscle also assist in breathing but are located deep within the chest wall. For Power Breathing, the intercostals are supplementary, with the internal intercostals aiding in controlling a long, steady exhalation by controlling the contraction of the ribs and chest cavity.

Rectus Abdominis

The rectus abdominis muscle is commonly known as the "abs". This muscle relaxes and expands during inhalation, tenses during condensing and contracts during exhalation. In Power Breathing, the elasticity of the diaphragm and the rectus abdominis is critical. They work together to take oxygen into the body yet function antagonistically, with one contracting while the other relaxes or expands and vice versa.

Transversus Abdominis

The transversus abdominis is the deepest abdominal muscle in the belly. The primary function of the transversus abdominis is to protect the major joints and the nervous system during movement and stabilize the body during lifting movements. In Power Breathing the transversus abdominis works hand-in-hand with the rectus abdominis to build power and inner force in the core of the torso.

The Pelvic Diaphragm

The pelvic diaphragm (also commonly known as pelvic floor) spans the area beneath the pelvic cavity, separating the pelvic cavity from the perineal region that lies below it. It consists of the levator ani and the coccygeus muscles. The main functions of the pelvic diaphragm are to support the organs in the pelvic cavity (the bladder, small intestine, colon, and uterus (in women)), and control continence. For Power Breathing, the pelvic diaphragm provides stability during inhalation, intensifies the inner pressure during the condensing process and contributes to speed control during exhalation.

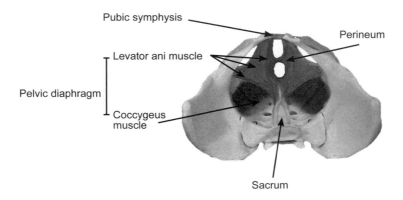

Putting it all Together

While holding the breath after inhalation, keep all of the muscles in a neutral condition (neither intentionally contracted nor relaxed). Focus on filling the cavities of the torso with air. During the initial condensing stage, tighten the transversus abdominis muscles on the side of the trunk. While holding the breath, tighten the abs (rectus abdominis). During the intense condensing stage, tense all of the muscles of the lower trunk including the rectus abdominis in the center, transversus abdominis on the side, the pelvic diaphragm on the bottom. Simultaneously, close your throat to prevent air from escaping.

THE ROLE OF OXYGEN

The essential function of breathing is to deliver oxygen to where it is needed in the body and remove carbon dioxide waste. Each breath that we take in is made up of about 78% nitrogen, 21% oxygen and small amounts of carbon dioxide and other gases. In a normal breath, we exhale about 4-5% carbon dioxide and about 16-17% oxygen as well as water vapor and other gases. As you can see from these numbers, only about 4-5% of the oxygen inhaled in the average breath is used by the body and the rest is simply lost back into the air around us.

However, the amount of oxygen retained by the body varies according to your fitness level and energy usage. By taking long deep breaths, controlling your exhalation and increasing your breathing capacity, you can take advantage of a greater percentage of the oxygen your body is already taking in.

How the Body Uses Oxygen

When you inhale, air rushes into the lungs where it is warmed, moistened and cleansed by the upper airways. In the lungs, it passes into smaller and smaller tube-like structures called bronchioles until it reaches tiny sacs called alveoli. Capillaries carry blood past the alveoli and the alveoli enrich the blood with oxygen. Once in the bloodstream, oxygen is carried by hemoglobin in the red blood cells. The blood exits the lungs through blood vessels and enters the left side of the heart, where it is pumped out to the rest of the body.

A series of arteries deliver the oxygenated blood to the cells of the body, once again reaching networks of small capillaries that deliver the oxygen to individual cells. The cells have an energy centers, called mitochondria, that convert the oxygen to energy that powers the cells. In the process, carbon dioxide is released and transferred to the hemoglobin in the blood, which returns it via a network of veins through the heart and lungs. When you exhale, this carbon dioxide is released from the body.

Essential Oxygen

As demonstrated in the simple explanation above, oxygen is essential to our bodies at the most basic cellular level. We can go weeks without food and days without water, but without oxygen, we can survive mere minutes. Allowing the bloodstream to absorb sufficient amounts of oxygen from every breath we take is an essential part of a healthy lifestyle and one of the primary aims of Power Breathing.

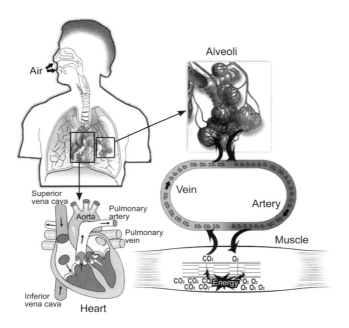

When you inhale, air rushes into the lungs and reaches tiny sacs called alveoli. The alveoli enrich the blood with oxygen. Hemoglobin then carries oxygen to individual cells via the left side of the heart and networks of small capillaries. In the cells, energy centers called mitochondria convert the oxygen into energy. In the process, carbon dioxide is released.

3

POWER BREATHING BASICS

THE GOLDEN CENTER

In the middle of the body, there is an imaginary space called the Golden Center, which is the center of your inner energy. To locate your Golden Center, it is important to first make space within your body. Your body is already filled with organs, vessels, lymph nodes, fluids, membranes, bones, muscles and air. Each has its own place and for optimal health, each requires enough space to reside, function or circulate. Blood moves through blood vessels; oxygen enters the lungs; the organs reside in the cavities of the torso. The space in which each of these essential elements resides or circulates is as important as the element itself. If blood cannot circulate freely, we suffer a heart attack or stroke. If our oxygen supply is restricted, our muscles, organs and brain suffer. If the cavities in our torso are cramped or crowded, our organs press on top of each other or collapse, impairing their function.

What keeps the space within the body functional is the structure of the body: skeletal and muscular. Similarly, our inner energy needs space to flourish and this space is the Golden Center.

BREATHING ROOM ◉

On The Useful Void

Lao Tzu, a philosopher and a mythical figure of ancient China in the 6th century BC, believed that emptiness is the source of all creation: without hinges, a door is useless; without an axle, the cart cannot roll; without a womb, there is no new life.

Tao Te Ching: Chapter 11

Thirty spokes join at a hub,
Without the hole, the cart makes no move.
From clay is moulded a pot,
Without the hollow, the pot has no use.
With wood is built a house,
Without the empty room, no dwelling is possible.
We make what is,
We use what is not.

道 德 經 ： 第 十 一 章
三 十 輻 ， 共 一 轂 ， 當 其 無 ， 有 車 之 月
埏 埴 以 為 器 ， 當 其 無 ， 有 器 之 用 。
鑿 戶 牖 以 為 室 ， 當 其 無 ， 有 室 之 用 。
故 有 之 以 為 利 ， 無 之 以 為 用 。

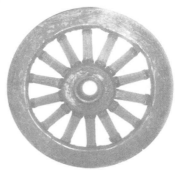

The Wheel of force and the golden center.

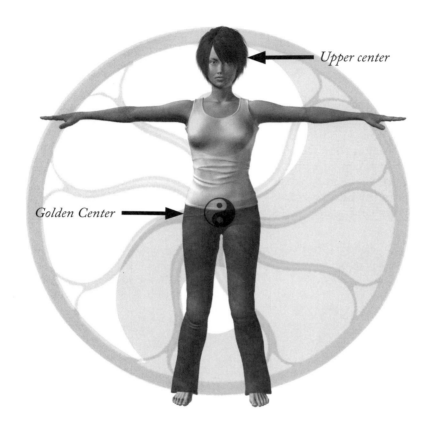

Upper center

Golden Center

Centering for Power

The center is the source of life force. In Power Breathing, the center of the body, called the Golden Center, is the focus of attention. By aligning your body naturally and shifting your attention from your brain to your lower belly, your biorhythm becomes calmer. After 3 deep breaths, the mind begins to be less active. After 10 breaths, the body begins to resume its natural balance. When your center becomes the calmest part of your body, the surrounding organs become more active which raises your body temperature and increases blood circulation. The hollower the center becomes, the deeper your breathing is. The usefulness of the center is its emptiness and calmness: the emptiness for receiving new energy, the calmness for freeing the busy mind.

Energy Centers

The center is like a home where we return to rest and recharge our energy. It brings our physical and mental senses back to awareness of who we are. It also provides us with a kinetic point that we can count on in movement. Without a sense of center, parts of the body may move independently, without integration. Then our body gets lost, just as our mind wanders when we lack mental focus. Having a sense of center is precious for our life, so it is named the Golden Center, signifying a precious home of the mind and body.

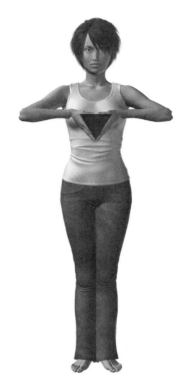

Find your middle energy center by bringing your fingertips together in front of your chest.

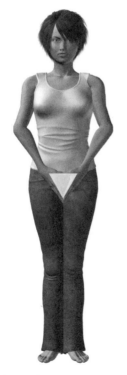

Find your lower energy center by bringing your fingertips together in front of your pelvis.

The Golden Center is where our focus comes from and where it returns to. It is the center of our confidence and efficiency. It can eventually free us from physical hindrance, mental blocks and spiritual stagnation. Just as our feelings affect our performance, physical awkwardness or discomfort profoundly impacts our self-perception. That's why having a sense of being centered is critical in breathing, moving and living.

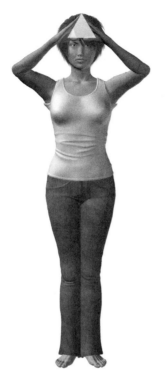

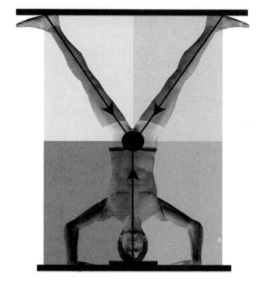

Find your upper energy center by bringing your fingertips together in front of your forehead.

Energy flows toward the Golden Center no matter position the body is in.

The Golden Center is just above the bladder in the upper middle of the pelvic cavity. It is a kind of imaginary reproductive place where new energy is created and stored, like an energy womb.

Out of the three energy centers in the body (the upper, middle and lower centers), the Golden Center (lower energy center) is the base. The middle center is on the centerline of the body, between the nipples. The upper center is between the eyes and is also known as the third eye.

The lower center is the seat of all physical force of the body. The middle center is the seat of emotional and mental energy. The upper center is the seat of the spiritual being.

The Feet: Foundation of the Body

The feet are the foundation for posture. From the middle point between the feet rises a vertical line that connects and stabilizes the three energy centers.

If the feet are the major base for the body, each energy center has its own minor base: the perineum is the minor base for the lower energy center, the solar plexus for the middle energy center, and the philtrum for the upper energy center. The minor bases are approximately 3 inches below their respective energy centers. The strength and elasticity of the muscles in the minor bases are important for Power Breathing because they support the tension and relaxation of the muscles of the respective centers. A strong base facilitates a sound hub for energy flow.

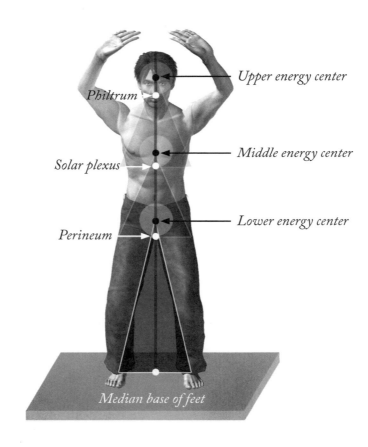

Philtrum

Upper energy center

Solar plexus

Middle energy center

Perineum

Lower energy center

Median base of feet

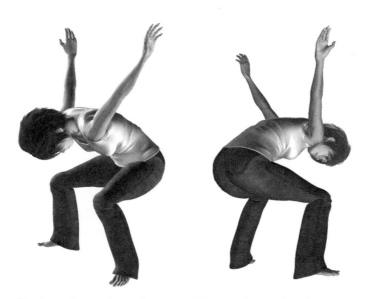

The buttocks are the synchronizers. They coordinate the left and right, upward and downward, and forward and backward movements.

Synchronize the Body

There are seven sections of the body to synchronize for generating maximum power: the feet and legs, the lower abdomen, the chest, the arms and the head. The feet and legs are the mobilizers and stabilizers of the torso. The lower abdomen is the energy reservoir. The chest is the distribution center for oxygen and blood. The arms are movement guides. The head is the command center. When these seven parts work in harmony, we are free of inner conflict and can experience the unconscious unity of mind and body.

If you try to assemble these separate pieces each time you make a new movement, it is hard to synchronize them. Instead, focus on moving the Golden Center, and everything else follows naturally. By focusing on one point, you will find that complicated movements become less complicated. Simply let the center of your body lead and the other parts follow. Distribute your energy from the center to accommodate each movement, so that your energy travels from the center to the terminals instead of the reverse.

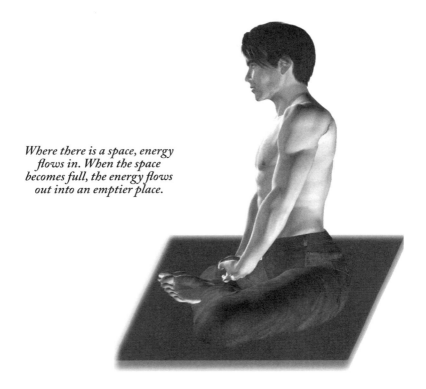

Where there is a space, energy flows in. When the space becomes full, the energy flows out into an emptier place.

FOLLOW THE RHYTHMIC FLOW

Breathing is not a static activity. Even when your breath appears very calm externally, your internal organs are constantly working to receive, distribute and expel the components of the air. The dynamic nature of breathing becomes evident when you move to belly breathing and even more evident in Power Breathing.

Power Breathing is a dynamic method of breathing which is most effective when you are able to sense and follow the rhythmic flow of your body. Rather than forcing your breath in and out, try to communicate with your body and find your own best rhythm. Just as waves break on the beach at consistent intervals, your breath naturally comes into the body and leaves the body at consistent intervals. Let the air enter the lungs like water filling a pond. When the breathing is right, there are no lungs and no belly, but just you, breathing in and breathing out.

On the next page are suggested Power Breathing patterns. Experiment with them to find your own best rhythmic flow.

DURATION CONTROL & INTENSITY LEVEL

We've talked a great deal about control during Power Breathing, but if you are not experienced in breathing exercises, it may be difficult at first to balance the duration of each segment of the breath. Below are some suggestions for you to experiment with when practicing the exercises that follow in Chapters 4 through 8. Always begin at a comfortable level, usually Level One, when starting a new exercise. Practice for one minute at a time to start. As you progress, move from one level to the next without skipping any levels. The advanced levels can be quite strenuous and some practitioners may never reach these levels.

WARNING: These are suggested guidelines only. You should proceed at your own pace and use common sense. Attempting levels beyond your ability may result in shortness of breath, dizziness, or fainting. If you feel discomfort during any exercise, stop immediately and return to your normal breathing.

Level One: Beginner
Inhale for 3 seconds
Hold for 2 seconds
Exhale for 5 seconds
Total 6 repetitions per minute
Intensity level: MILD

Level Two: Beginner
Inhale for 3 seconds
Condense for 2 seconds
Exhale for 5 seconds
Total 6 Repetitions per minute
Intensity level: MILD

Level Three: Intermediate
Inhale for 4 seconds
Condense for 4 seconds
Exhale for 4 seconds
Total 5 Repetitions per minute
Intensity level: MODERATE

Level Four: Intermediate
Inhale for 4 seconds
Condense for 5 seconds
Exhale for 6 seconds
Total 4 Repetitions per minute
Intensity level: MODERATE

Level Five: Advanced
Inhale for 5 seconds
Condense for 5 seconds
Exhale for 10 seconds
Total 3 Repetitions per minute
Intensity level: STRENUOUS

Level Six: Advanced
Inhale for 10 seconds
Condense for 5 seconds
Exhale for 15 seconds
Total 2 Repetitions per minute
Intensity level: STRENUOUS
* CAUTION: Only if you are ready.

Level Seven: Expert
Inhale for 15 seconds
Exhale for 5 seconds
Condense for 5 seconds
 Release for 15 seconds
Total 3 Repetitions per 2 minutes
Intensity level: CHALLENGING
**CAUTION: Only if you are ready.

* Release is another term for exhaling and is commonly used when describing exhalation after the condensing stage.

A Word about Intensity

Before you begin to practice the exercises of Power Breathing, it is important to understand the level of intensity that is right for your body, especially in the condensing stage.

There are several interrelated elements that affect your breathing including duration, frequency, speed and depth and they vary based on your physical and psychological condition. Intensity, however, is generally independent of the other elements. It is more relevant to how much intentional muscular force you apply to the process of inhalation or exhalation. By contracting and expanding your muscles, you can adjust the degree of intensity of your breathing. You may inhale with a short, fast, shallow and intense breath and exhale with a long, slow, deep and gentle breath. Generally, it is good to practice a long, slow, deep and moderate inhalation, a moderate to intense condensing, and a very long, slow, deep exhalation.

However, each intensity level has appropriate applications. During mild intensity, similar to your regular breathing, you are conscious of belly breathing and hold the muscles of the diaphragm and belly during a brief pause between stages. For moderate intensity, inhale and tense the inner muscles to create inner pressure from the chest to the Solar Plexus. For strenuous intensity, press the Golden Ball down toward the umbilicus and the Golden Center. For challenging intensity, press the Golden Ball down toward the perineum.

For safety, practice condensing progressively. If you are new to breathing exercises or recovering from time off due to an injury or illness, stay below 5 on the intensity scale. If you are a professional athlete, pilot, deep water diver, or climber, you may push beyond 8 on the scale. For general practitioners, I recommend staying between intensity levels 2 and 8.

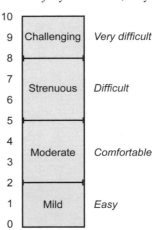

Intensity chart

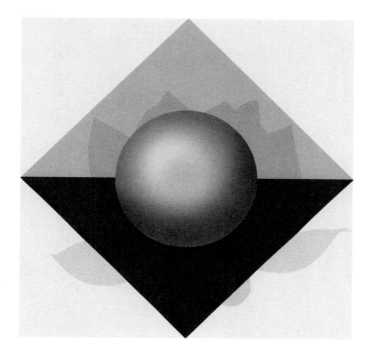

3 EXERCISES
FOR CENTERING AND RHYTHMIC FLOW

There are simple exercises you can do to establish the elements necessary for Power Breathing: stabilize your stance and posture, create more room in your body, center your energy, and control your internal rhythm. The Sunrise Breathing, Awakening Lotus and Diamond Breathing exercises on the following pages will help you prepare for more strenuous Power Breathing exercises by relaxing and expanding your inner muscles, integrating the parts of your body as a whole, and bringing your body and mind together, like two wheels working together to move a cart.

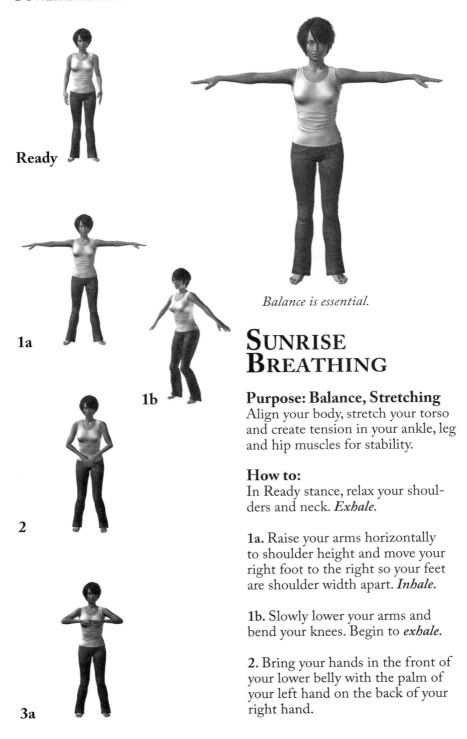

Ready

1a

1b

2

3a

Balance is essential.

SUNRISE BREATHING

Purpose: Balance, Stretching
Align your body, stretch your torso and create tension in your ankle, leg and hip muscles for stability.

How to:
In Ready stance, relax your shoulders and neck. *Exhale.*

1a. Raise your arms horizontally to shoulder height and move your right foot to the right so your feet are shoulder width apart. *Inhale.*

1b. Slowly lower your arms and bend your knees. Begin to *exhale.*

2. Bring your hands in the front of your lower belly with the palm of your left hand on the back of your right hand.

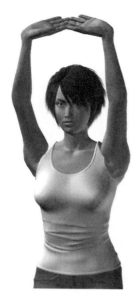

3c

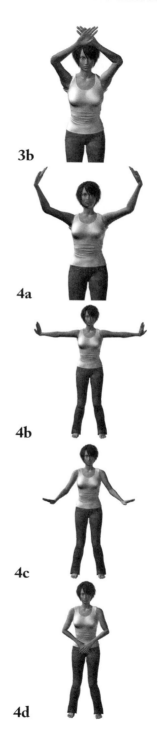

3b

4a

4b

4c

4d

3a. Raise both hands, palms down, slowly to your chest. Begin to *inhale*.

3b. Let your hands pass your face, continuing to *inhale*.

3c. Stretch your hands and arms all the way above your head and pause here for 3 seconds. Continue to *inhale*.

4a. Gently lower your hands to the sides, palms outward. Begin to *exhale*.

4b. Keep your wrists bent and continue to *exhale* as you lower your arms.

4c. Continue to lower your hands and tense your belly muscles to push the air out of the body.

4d. Bringing your hands to your lower belly, *hold* the breath for 3 seconds. From here, return to normal breathing in ready posture.

Repeat Sunrise Breathing 10 times.

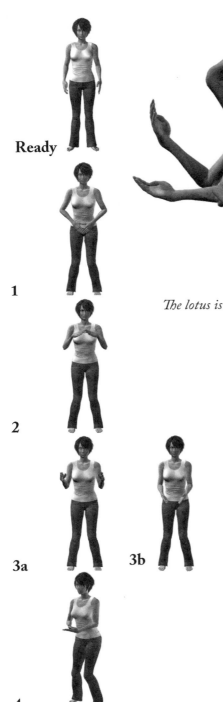

Ready

1

2

3a   3b

4

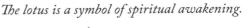

The lotus is a symbol of spiritual awakening.

AWAKENING LOTUS

Purpose: Toning The Lungs
Gently work the lungs in a slow even rhythm. Keep your elbows close to your body to assist in controlling the chest muscles.

How to:
In Ready stance, relax your shoulders and neck. *Exhale.*

1. Bend your knees and bring your hands in front of your lower belly.

2. Raise your hands along the median line slowly and *inhale*. Pause your hands in front of the chest and *hold* your breath for 3 seconds.

3a & b. Begin to *exhale* and bring your hands outward and downward in a circular motion.

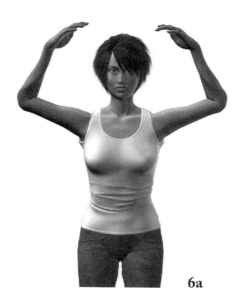

6a

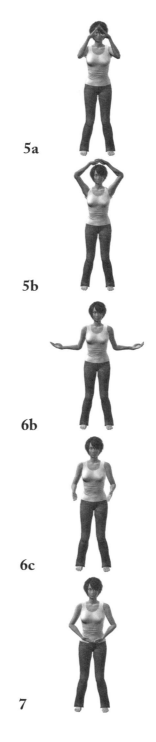

5a

5b

6b

6c

7

4. In front of your lower belly, rest the back of your right hand on top of your left palm. *Hold* your breath for 3 seconds.

5a & b. Begin to *inhale* and raise your hands along the median line (with palms down) to your face and then above your head. Stop and *hold* the breath for 3 seconds.

6a, b & c. Open your hands to the sides and begin to *exhale*. Slowly lower your hands. Imagine you are pulling an elastic from both ends and feel the weight of your arms through the inner muscles of your chest.

7. In front of your lower belly, rest the back of your right hand on top of your left palm (palms up). *Hold* your breath for 3 seconds. From here, return to normal breathing in ready posture.

Repeat Awakening Lotus Breathing 10 times.

* If you feel short of breath, reduce the length of each breath until you feel comfortable.

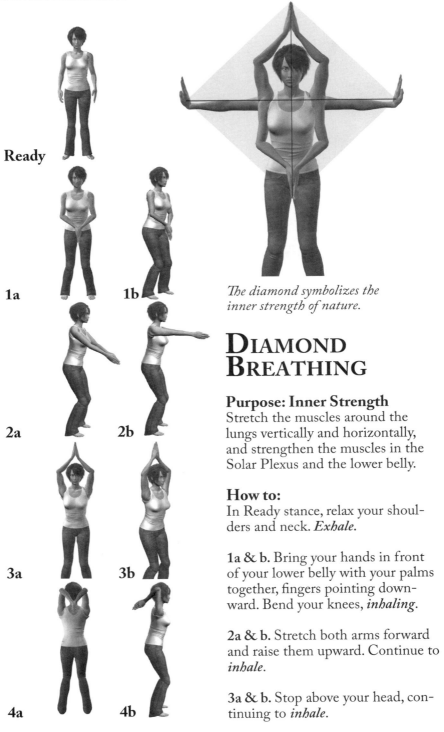

Ready

1a   **1b**

2a   **2b**

3a   **3b**

4a   **4b**

The diamond symbolizes the inner strength of nature.

DIAMOND BREATHING

Purpose: Inner Strength
Stretch the muscles around the lungs vertically and horizontally, and strengthen the muscles in the Solar Plexus and the lower belly.

How to:
In Ready stance, relax your shoulders and neck. *Exhale.*

1a & b. Bring your hands in front of your lower belly with your palms together, fingers pointing downward. Bend your knees, *inhaling.*

2a & b. Stretch both arms forward and raise them upward. Continue to *inhale.*

3a & b. Stop above your head, continuing to *inhale.*

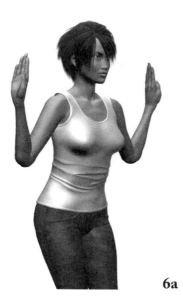

6a

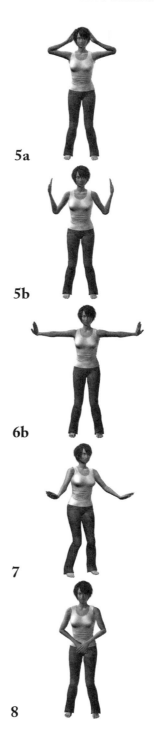

5a

5b

6b

7

8

4a & b. Lower your hands to your spine and continue to *inhale*.

5a. Open your elbows to both sides, continuing to *inhale*.

5b. Lower your elbows, turn your palms outward, and continue to *inhale*.

6a & b. Slowly push your hands outward and begin to *exhale*. Contract the muscles of your upper belly and regulate the force of exhalation.

7. Slowly lower your hands in a circular motion toward your lower belly. Continue to *exhale*. Contract the muscles in your lower belly.

8. *Hold* the breath for a moment and contract the lower belly muscles further. From here, return to normal breathing in ready posture.

Repeat Diamond Breathing 10 times.

* If you feel short of breath, reduce the length of each breath until you feel comfortable.

PHILOSOPHY

Five Elements of Life Force

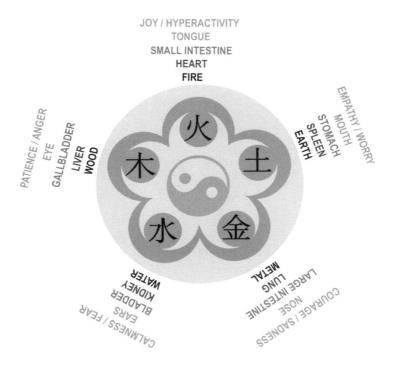

In Traditional Chinese Medicine (TCM) the natural elements of Fire, Earth, Metal, Water and Wood correspond to the organs, meridians, emotions and senses. Each element or force generates or creates the next element in the sequence and similarly, each organ supports a related organ. For example, the kidney supports the liver and the liver supports the heart. The elements and organs also perform a regulating function on other elements, with the kidney controlling the heart in the same way that water controls fire. TCM practitioners use these relationships to assist in diagnosing and correcting imbalances of energy (Ki or Chi) in the body. As you practice Power Breathing, keep the relationships of nature, our bodies and life energy in mind. Soon, you will feel your energy increasing, your connectedness to nature enhanced and your body at one with your mind.

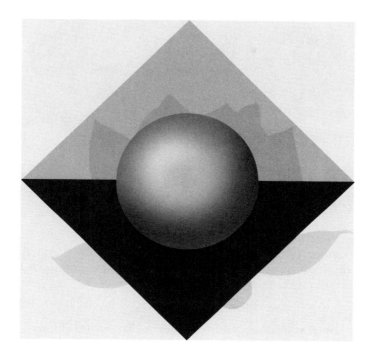

EXERCISES
FOR RESTING THE ORGANS

Because we walk upright, our organs sit on top of each other, which can lead to one organ pressing on another over time. By practicing the Sleeping Turtle and Waking Alligator postures on the following pages, you can give your organs a rest.

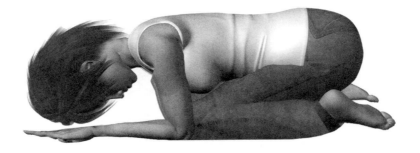

SLEEPING TURTLE

Purpose: Resting the Organs
This is a unique exercise for releasing the stress of normal gravity on the organs. Think of the organs as apples, peaches, grapes and pears hanging freely from branches as you rest.

How to:
Kneel as low as you comfortably can on your knees and elbows with your palms on the floor and your elbows gently pressing against your knees. Hold your head slightly above the floor. Let your torso rest like the roof of a house. Relax your shoulders and neck. *Inhale* and *exhale* freely a few times.

When you are ready, slowly *inhale*, filling the belly. The fullness should lift the torso like a submarine floating above the water. *Hold* for 3-8 seconds and tense your muscles gently to increase the inner force in your torso.

Slowly *exhale* and let your torso sink while controlling your belly muscles.

Repeat 10 times.

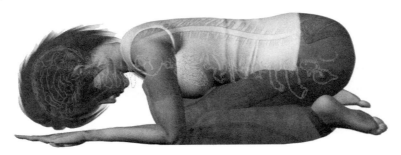

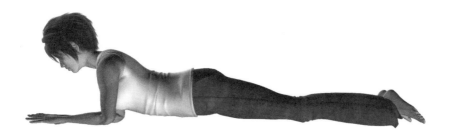

WAKING ALLIGATOR

Purpose: Releasing Tension in the Pelvic Cavity

This is an active resting exercise for organs in the pelvic cavity. Elevate your torso approximately 45 degrees so that the organs rest diagonally. Let the belly lift your body gently during *inhalation*.

How to:

Lie on your stomach. Raise your upper body, supporting it with your elbows. Rest your body primarily on your pelvis and elbows.

Inhale and let the belly lift your body gently. When the belly is full, *hold* for 3-8 seconds.

Exhale gently and slowly.
Feel your body weight on your belly.
Reluctantly let your body sink.

Shift your body weight toward your elbows and complete your exhalation.

Repeat 10 times.

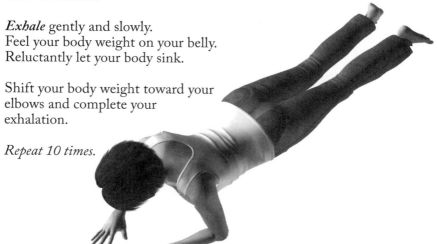

KEYS OF POWER BREATHING

5 Types of Power Breathing:

Gentle Breathing for suppleness
Explosive Breathing for expansion
Steady Breathing for stability
Staccato Breathing for vitality
Healing Breathing for restoration

3 Power Breathing Basics:

1) *Inhale*: Expand your belly and fill the lungs with oxygen.
2) *Condense:* Tense all of the muscles to increase the inner force.
3) *Exhale:* Relax the diaphragm and distribute the energy.

Benefits of Power Breathing:

Some of the physical and mental benefits include:

- stronger heart and lungs
- strong, supple muscles and healthy ligaments
- more flexibility, coordination, and balance
- enhanced awareness, physical confidence and mental concentration
- natural weight control
- boosted energy level and sense of well-being

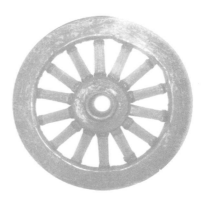

4

GENTLE BREATHING

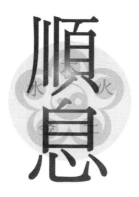

順息

순식

Soon-shik

INTENSITY LEVEL: MILD

Expand the Belly Muscles

Power Breathing begins with expansion of the belly muscles to create space in the abdominal cavity into which the diaphragm can descend (contract). This in turn creates more space in the chest cavity, where the lungs then expand and air enters into the body. Exhalation takes place in reverse. Gentle Breathing increases the suppleness and strength of the muscles of the belly and diaphragm. In your daily breathing practice, gentle breathing is a good way to begin and end a session.

Diaphragm Exercise

The distance that the diaphragm travels is important for our overall health. The more it can contract (descend during inhaling), the more it can relax (ascend during exhaling). And the more it can relax, the higher it travels up into the lungs forcing the lungs to expel more carbon dioxide from the body. Gentle Breathing progressively enhances the elasticity of the diaphragm.

HOLDING THE BREATH

The purpose of holding the breath is to prolong and smooth the transitional process between the two opposing activities of inhalation and exhalation. Additionally, by holding the breath you are momentarily pausing and tensing the muscles of the belly and diaphragm (like an isometric exercise for the inner muscles), creating tension. Holding the breath is a good way to develop the muscular strength and elasticity essential to a strong, pain-free torso.

Breath Holding Methods

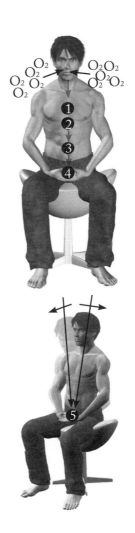

1. Chest Holding
Inhale for 2 seconds, stop the breath and bring your awareness to your chest. *Hold* for 3 seconds, and then *exhale*. Repeat 5 times.

2. Solar Plexus Holding
Inhale for 3 seconds, stop the breath and bring your awareness to your Solar Plexus. *Hold* for 3 seconds, and then *exhale*.
Repeat 5 times.

3. Umbilicus Holding
Inhale for 4 seconds, stop the breath and bring your awareness to your umbilicus. *Hold* for 3 seconds, and then *exhale*. Repeat 5 times.

4. Golden Center Holding
Inhale for 5 seconds, stop the breath and bring your awareness to your lower abdomen. *Hold* for 3 seconds, and then *exhale*.
Repeat 5 times.

LOCATION SPOTTING TIP:
You can tilt your body slightly forward or backward to feel the tension in the Golden Center (5).

GENTLE BREATHING EFFECTS

Gentle Breathing is simply breathing in and out, focusing your mind on the process. Initially you will be very conscious of the specifics, such as how much to expand and contract the belly muscles and how long to hold. Don't worry about it. Just breathe in, hold, and breathe out according to your instinct. By simply repeating the process over and over, you'll find your own best method. If you feel uncomfortable, experiment until you feel comfortable. After ten repetitions, you will slowly begin to stop thinking about breathing and FEEL YOUR BREATHING. Soon you will just breathe without splitting your mind-body unity. You will become one.

The following are some potential benefits of Gentle Breathing:

1. Increased awareness of your body.

2. Increased pressure in the belly which stimulates the function of the organs such as the large intestine, kidney, bladder, spleen, small intestine, and reproductive organs.

3. Enhanced digestion.

4. Increased capacity of the lungs and heart. Regular gentle breathing boosts blood circulation and oxygen delivery to the cells which increases the body's energy level.

5. Cleansing of toxins in the body, through longer slower exhalation.

6. Calming effect on the autonomous nervous system. Regular gentle breathing lowers blood pressure.

7. Improved concentration, muscle relaxation, and mental composure due to improved oxygen supply to the brain and body.

SITTING BREATHING

On the Floor

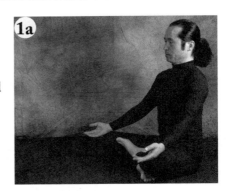

1a. Sit with your legs crossed.
* If you have difficulty in folding your legs, sit with your legs stretched (**1b**) or with your legs bent in a diamond shape (**1c**).

2. Keep your back, neck, and head aligned along your centerline. Gaze about 45 degrees downward with a sense of looking inward.

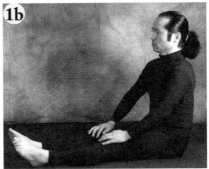

3. Relax your shoulders and arms. Place your right hand on top of your upper foot with the palm facing upward and let the back of your left hand rest on your right palm. Bring the tips of your thumbs together.

4. Expand your belly and *inhale* through your nose for 3 seconds. Hold for 3 seconds. *Exhale* through your nose for 3 seconds, letting your belly muscles contract naturally.

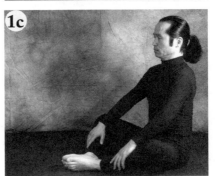

POWER TIP:

While holding your breath, contract the pelvic diaphragm. This creates upward tension in the lower stomach and natural contraction of the abdominal muscles. If this is too hard, don't worry, we'll do it again in later exercises.

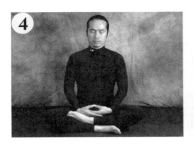

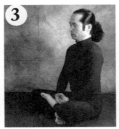

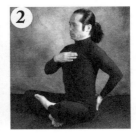

SITTING BREATHING
DETAILED INSTRUCTION

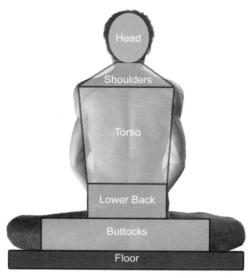

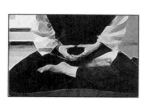

Full lotus posture

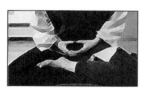

Half lotus posture

Each part of your body is firmly but gently in its place and there is no need to tense your muscles. Then, your body becomes a stable house in which your mind can be free of distractions.

POSTURE

Gentle Breathing can be done while standing, seated or lying down, however, sitting is a good way to develop your posture and stay mindfully alert during your practice. You may cross your legs in the full lotus or half-lotus position or any comfortable position.

When you sit, imagine resting your buttocks on the earth itself. Align your spine and torso perpendicular to the earth and feel your spine resting firmly on your buttocks. When your spine is firmly rooted and your lower back is stable, you can easily relax your shoulders and neck.

Similarly, let your arms flow from your shoulders without tension and your hands rest naturally in front of you.

A stable posture and relaxed muscles enable you to breathe naturally and deeply. An unstable posture and tense muscles result in short and shallow breathing. Recheck your posture periodically during your practice to be sure you are relaxed and centered.

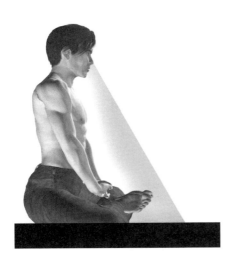

EYES

You can keep your eyes open or closed, depending on your personal preference. If you keep your eyes open, don't let your vision wander. Try to focus on a single spot in the near distance. Relax your eyelids and look downward at a 45 degree angle. Or simply look at the tip of your nose. Gradually your awareness will move from sight to inner consciousness.

If you close your eyes, do so gently and try to see your inner self.

HANDS AND FEET POSITIONS

Place your hands wherever you find most comfortable. Traditionally, in meditation and breathing exercises, the hands are placed in the lap with the right hand on the bottom and the left hand on top of it.

In Eastern philosophy, the hands are placed according to the principle of Yin (weak) and Yang (powerful). In placing the hands, the right hand represents the Yang force so it is set down first as a powerful base. The left hand represents Yin and is placed on top of the right. The two thumbs are then held with their tips touching, representing the union of Yin and Yang. It is believed that Yin and Yang are two manifestations of the same energy and one cannot exist without the other, so the forces are not opponents but they complement each other. When you place

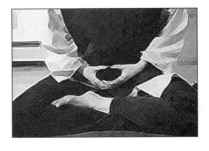

the tips of your thumbs together, imagine that the energy from the right (Yang) side and the energy from the left (Yin) side are communicating with each other.

You can take this concept one step further by crossing your legs with your right leg on the bottom and your left leg resting on it. Then place your right hand down on your crossed legs and your left hand on top. In this way your body is symmetrical and unified, making you feel more centered.

ALTERNATIVE METHOD

Sitting on a Chair

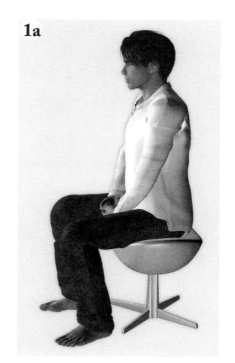

1a. If you find sitting on the floor difficult, sit on a chair. Relax your shoulders and arms, so your center of gravity sinks to your pelvis.

1b. Align your tailbone (a), spine (b) and head (c) vertically.

1c. Imagine that your torso and shoulders rest on the base of your hips, and your neck and head sit on your shoulders. When your torso and head feel anchored and supported, the muscles in the body can relax.

2. Expand your belly and create space as you *inhale*. When the belly is fully expanded, *hold* for 3 seconds. *Exhale* slowly, contracting the belly muscles.

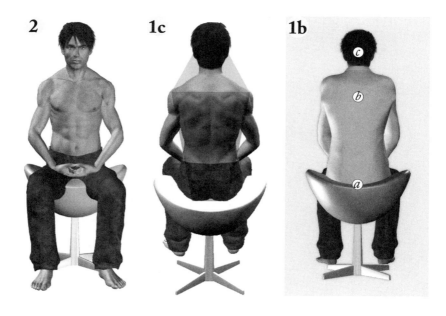

5

EXPLOSIVE BREATHING

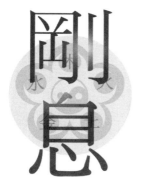

剛息

강식

Gang-shik

Condensing the Air

Explosive Breathing is a process of condensing the inhaled oxygen downward to the Golden Center, then distributing it to the organs, the limbs and the head.

The goal of Explosive Breathing is to create concentrated force for inner tension and relaxation.

Effects:

1) Increased circulation
2) Total upper body exercise
3) Increased inner power

Explosive Breathing Types:

1) Gentle Method
2) Soft Method
3) Dynamic Method
4) Kneeling Method

FIVE STEP BREATHING - OVERVIEW ◐

Five Step Breathing consists of one inhalation, one holding and three exhalation stages. After practicing Three Step Breathing - inhalation, condensing and exhalation for at least 3 months, try moving on to five step breathing to further expand your capacity to hold the breath and lengthen your exhalation with controlled force. Five step breathing is challenging, so be flexible and adapt the intensity and duration to your ability level.

Purpose: Intense Control of Inner Force

How to:

Inhale deeply and hold your breath firmly. Start the initial condensing gently with steady intensity and pace, then intensely condense the air. Finally release the tension through an explosive exhalation. Five step breathing is a good way to prepare for the more intense Power Breathing exercises that follow.

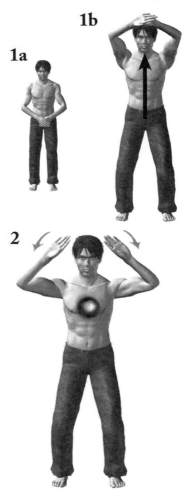

Step 1: Inhalation

Put your hands in front of the lower belly overlapped and *exhale* deeply (1a). Raise your hands above your head and *inhale* deeply (1b).

Step 2: Holding

When your hands arrive above your head, *hold* your breath for 3 seconds. Slowly drop your hands to chest height at the side of your body while continuing to *hold* your breath.

Step 3: Initial Condensing

The initial condensing is the beginning of forced *exhalation* (3a). As you lower your arms, contract your belly muscles and visualize compressing the air from the chest through the solar plexus and umbilicus down to the Golden Center (3b). When you've exhaled about 2/3 of the way, your hands should arrive in front of the Golden Center. *Hold* your breath for 2-3 seconds there.

Step 4: Intense Condensing

Intensively tighten all the core muscles (rectus abdominis, transversus abdominis, intercostals, pelvic diaphragm and diaphragm) while pushing both hands upward (4). At this time you will have a natural spurt or short forceful expulsion (*exhalation*) of air through your nose or mouth. Keep pushing your hands upward slowly but forcefully while exhaling (5a).

Step 5: Explosion

Explosion takes place when your hands reach your chest (5a). At this point let the condensed air in the body explode and let your hands go as you finish *exhaling* (5b). Then, repeat steps 1-5.

* Explosion is a type of intense release.

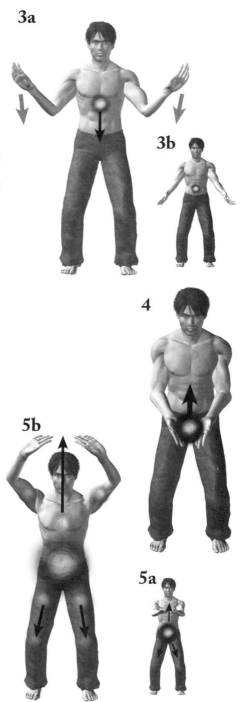

EXPLOSIVE BREATHING

General Method

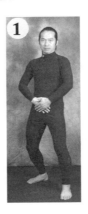

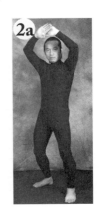

1. Stand with your feet shoulder width apart and your hands in front of the lower belly. *Exhale.*

2a. Quickly raise your hands above your head and *inhale.*

2b-c. Lower your hands in an outward circular motion to position 1 and *exhale.*

3a-c. Repeat steps 2a to 2c.

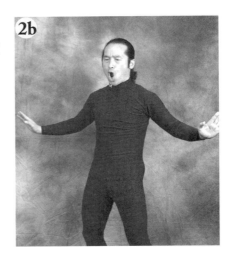

4. Raise your hands above your head and *inhale* to your maximum, then *hold* for 2 seconds.

5. While *holding* the breath, slowly lower your hands outward in a circular motion.

6. Begin to *exhale*, continuing to lower your hands while contracting the belly muscles and condensing from the chest down toward the Golden Center.

7. At the two thirds of your exhalation, when your hands arrive in front of the Golden Center, *hold* your breath for 2 seconds.

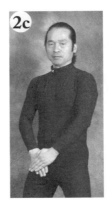

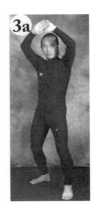

8. Abruptly and forcefully contract the muscles in the lowest belly and push both hands upward. At this time you will have a natural short forceful expulsion of air through your nose or mouth. Keep pushing your hands upward slowly but forcefully while *exhaling.*

Intensity chart of explosive breathing.

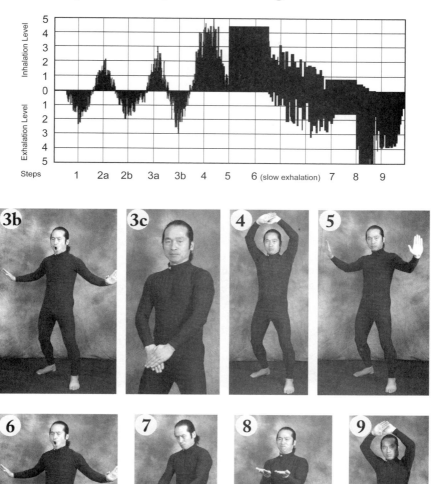

9. When your hands arrive at your chest level, *exhale* abruptly then raise your hands over your head and let go.

* Repeat steps 1-9 ten times. (For detailed instruction, see the following pages.)

EXPLOSIVE BREATHING
DETAILED INSTRUCTION

INHALATION

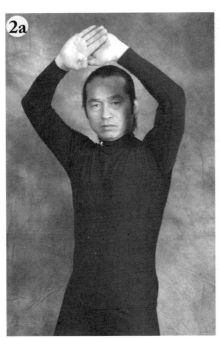

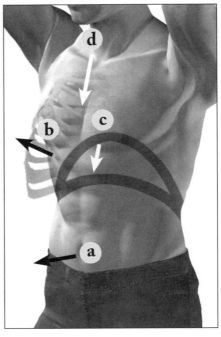

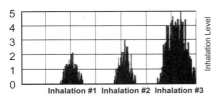

Progressive Intensity Escalation:

The intensity of the three initial inhalations is progressively stronger. The first is 1/3 of maximum intensity, the second is 2/3 and the last is at maximum intensity. Progressive intensity escalation is a way to safely and efficiently increase your inhalation capacity.

When you expand your belly (a) while raising your arms, the rib cage expands (b) and the diaphragm descends (c) making additional space in the thoracic cavity for more oxygen (d).

When the diaphragm contracts (while descending), it stimulates the organs beneath it such as the stomach, liver, gallbladder, spleen, and intestines, which activate blood circulation.

UPPER HOLDING

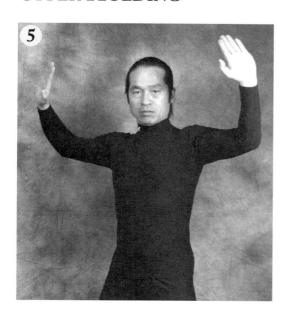

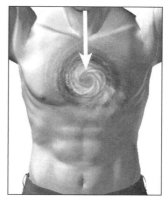

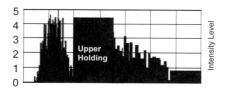

Upper Holding is Pre-condensing Stage:

The intensity of the inner pressure is constant during the Upper Holding stage. You should feel like there is a vacuum in your chest and belly region, like stillness before a tornado. Lower your arms to the sides very slowly feeling every inch of the movement.

The Upper Holding stage is a pre-condensing, transitional stage. During inhalation, the pressure in the chest is greater than the pressure in the belly. While holding, the pressure of the upper and lower body equalizes. Then during exhalation, the pressure in the belly becomes greater.

While holding the breath, visualize the air in your lungs flowing and whirling freely.

As you lower your arms slowly to the sides, imagine that you are shaping that air into a large light ball of air.

INITIAL CONDENSING

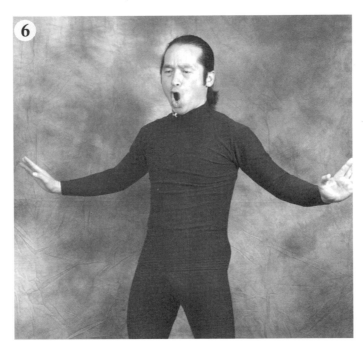

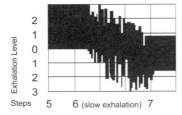

During exhalation, oxygen is carried into the blood stream. If your exhalation is too short, the oxygen taken in is wasted. Exhalation should occupy 2/3 of each breathing cycle. A long, slow exhalation helps your body absorb more oxygen and strengthens your inner muscles.

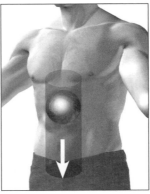

Constant Intensity Condensing:

Condensing is like a squeezing a snow ball to make it harder. The intensity of initial condensing should be applied at an even speed and pressure. Imagine that you are pressing a round ball of air slowly along a vertical cylinder in the body.

LOWER HOLDING

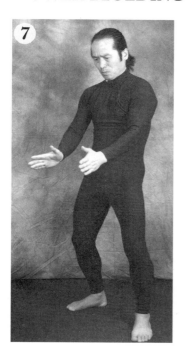

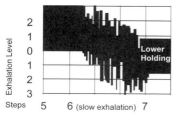

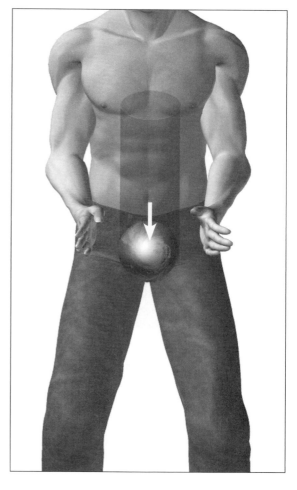

Sinking the Ball:

Lower Holding is a brief resting period to visualize dropping the condensed ball of air onto the pelvic floor. While holding the breath, imagine that you let go of the ball.

At the end of the initial condensing when your hands arrive in front of the Golden Center, hold your breath for 2 seconds. Let go of the imaginary air ball and drop it to the pelvic floor.

INTENSE CONDENSING

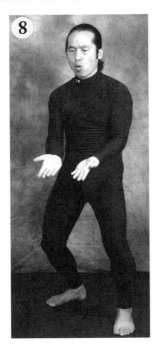

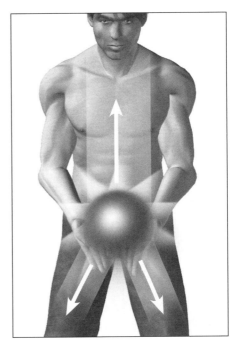

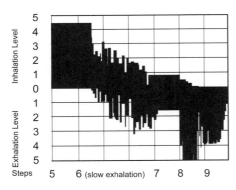

Intense Condensing:

Intense condensing takes place abruptly and forcefully immediately after the second holding stage. Contract all of the core muscles and slowly raise your hands like lifting a heavy weight.

Intense condensing increases circulation, as the intensity of the inner muscles reaches the maximum at this point and the blood pressure rises. Visualize your inner muscles squeezing the condensed air ball until it pops. When it pops, the energy from the ball penetrates every cell in the body. As your hands push upward moving the energy to the chest and head, another stream of energy travels to your feet.

* CAUTION: If you have high blood pressure, get dizzy/lightheaded or have a hernia, do not do this exercise. Instead, try the soft method on the next page.

ALTERNATIVE METHOD

Soft Method

1. Stand with your feet shoulder width apart and your hands in front of the lower belly. *Exhale*.

2a. Gently raise your hands above your head and *inhale*.

2b-c. Lower your hands outward in a circular motion and bring them to position 1. *Exhale*.

3a-c. Repeat steps 2a to 2c.

4a. Raise your hands above your head and *inhale* deeply.

4b. Slowly lower your hands outward in a circular motion and *exhale*.

4c. Continue to *exhale* and gently contract the muscles in the lower belly, pelvic floor and buttocks.

5. When your hands arrive at chest level, *hold* your breath for 2 seconds.

6. *Exhale*, raise your hands over your head and let go.

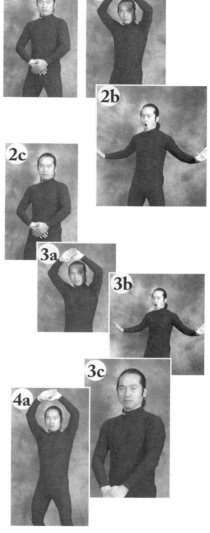

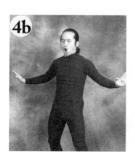
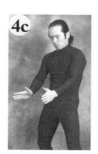
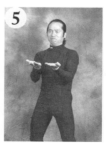
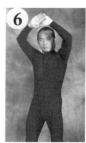

ALTERNATIVE METHOD

Dynamic Method

INTENSITY LEVEL: STRENUOUS

1. Stand with your feet shoulder width apart and your hands in front of the lower belly. *Exhale.*

2a-c. Move around freely, circling your arms outward. *Inhale* and *exhale* rapidly and forcefully twice.

3. Raise your hands above your head and *inhale* deeply.

4. Slowly lower your hands outward and condense while bending your knees. Contract all of your muscles and *exhale* intensely.

5. *Hold* your breath. Contract the muscles in your legs, hips, pelvic floor and belly. Very slowly straighten your legs and push your hands upward, like lifting a heavy weight, to create maximum pressure.

6a-b. When your hands arrive at chest level, *exhale* abruptly, raise your hands and let go.

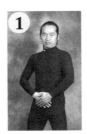
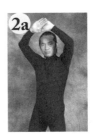
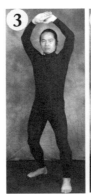
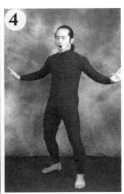
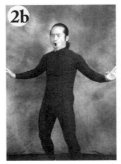
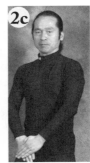
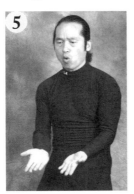
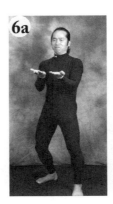
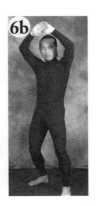

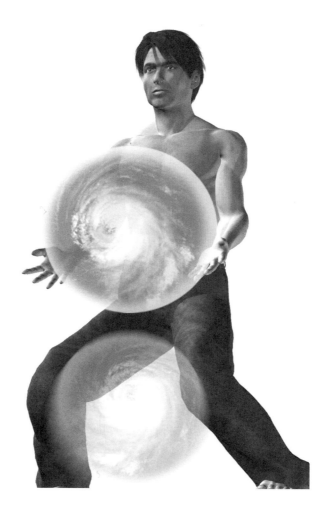

Visualize the Force: The dynamic method of Explosive Breathing aims to develop maximum muscle control for inner power. Imagine that you are lifting a heavy ball. For a strong stance, stand on the bottom bones of the big toes (the sesamoid bones) and the bottom of the inner heel. Squeeze your knees inward and contract the inner thigh muscles (gracilis) and buttock muscles (gluteus maximus), which naturally help the pelvic diaphragm contract. When these bases are constructed strongly, you can build maximum inner force.

KEY POINT ◑

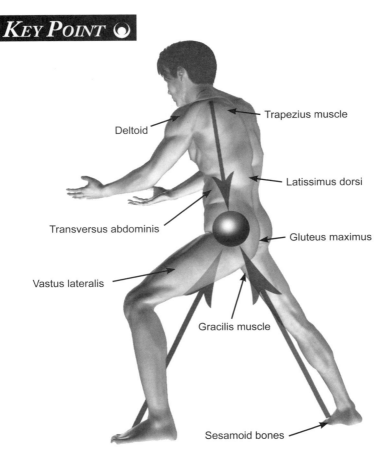

Trapezius muscle

Deltoid

Latissimus dorsi

Transversus abdominis

Gluteus maximus

Vastus lateralis

Gracilis muscle

Sesamoid bones

A well constructed stance has a perfectly aligned center that is supported by the correct placement of the feet, knees and hips. The center then becomes light and agile.

Your legs play an important part in creating stability and unifying your body in Power Breathing. Stand on the inside of the front of your feet (the sesamoid bones), rather than on your heels or flat on your soles. By standing on the inside edge of your feet, you create tension in your calves. Next, bend your knees slightly and squeeze your knees inward a bit, to create tension in your thighs. Finally, tilt your hips backward slightly when inhaling and tuck your hips in when condensing or exhaling. By using your hips actively in breathing, you are transferring the power of your legs to your torso and vice versa. Most importantly, keep your legs active during each exercise, drawing power up from the Earth.

ALTERNATIVE METHOD

Kneeling Method (for Posture Correction)

Kneeling Breathing reduces the pressure on your spine and diaphragm. Kneeling may be a painful posture initially, so you may need to put a blanket or mat on the floor to minimize discomfort. You may like this posture for a number of reasons:

1. Kneeling Breathing keeps your posture firm and strong by distributing your weight evenly on your knees, feet and buttocks.

2. Kneeling Breathing anchors your torso and corrects inappropriate posture, alleviating low back pain and shoulder and neck stiffness.

3. Kneeling Breathing reduces the pressure on your spine and diaphragm, which makes breathing easier and improves your breathing capacity.

4. Kneeling Breathing revitalizes the reproductive system.

5. Kneeling Breathing strengthens the joints, stretches the muscles in the legs and enhances the ability to control the muscles in the pelvic floor.

6. Kneeling Breathing stimulates acupoints in the legs and enhances circulation.

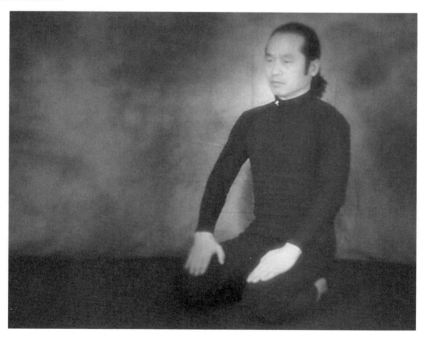

Kneeling Method

1. Kneel with your heels under your buttocks. Let your thighs rest on your lower legs and your buttocks on your heels. The whole body rests on the knees and ankles. Keep your knees slightly open for balance. Align your torso, neck and head.

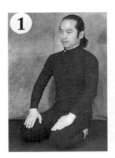
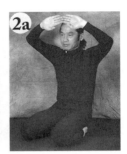

2a-c. Raise your hands above your head then lower them to the sides in a circular motion. *Inhale* and *exhale* rapidly & forcefully twice.

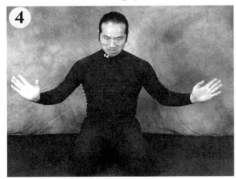

3. Raise your hands above your head and *inhale* deeply.

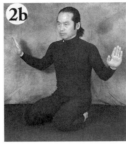
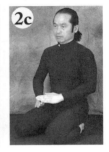

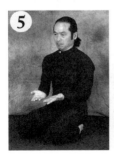
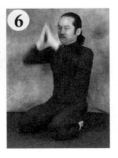
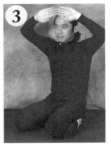

4. Slowly lower your hands in an outward circular motion and condense the air. Contract all of your muscles and *exhale* intensely.

5. *Hold* the breath. Raise your hands and contract the muscles in the lower belly and pelvic floor.

6. When your hands arrive at chest level, *exhale* abruptly, raise your hands and let go.

SOUND OF POWER ◑

EXPLOSIVE BREATHING WITH "*HEE-YAP-AHH!*"

While tensing the lower abdomen, vocalizing can help guide your exhalation. Start with "Hee", allowing the air to leak out of your mouth and then shout "Yap" while tensing the lower abdomen and finish with a releasing "Ahh".

1. Expand your belly fully and inhale. Exhale while forcefully saying "Hee" and gradually tightening the lower abdomen.
2. Shout "Yap" at the 2/3 point of the exhalation and hold. At this point, you should feel your throat close, your diaphragm still, and your buttocks and abs contract.

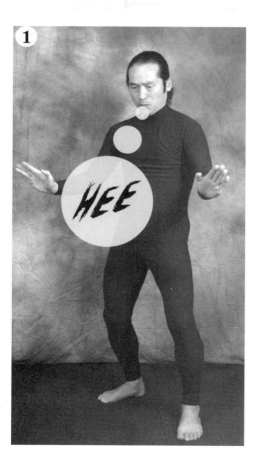

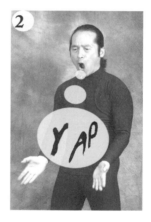

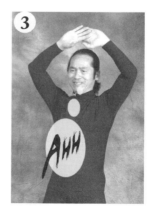

6

STEADY BREATHING

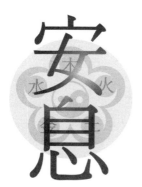

안 식

Ahn-shik

Equalize Intensity

Steady Breathing is an exercise to regulate the intensity and speed of the breath. The goal is to increase inner force by condensing and directing air from the throat (glottis) to the Golden Center. Force is applied evenly at a consistent speed to stabilize and strengthen the breathing channels.

Stabilize the Path

Steady Breathing focuses on an imaginary vertical path of the breath through the middle of the torso. Visualize moving the air from the throat down through the chest to the belly. Through active visualization and intentional muscular contraction of Steady Breathing, you are changing the condition of the inner environment of your body, increasing the internal pressure in the cavities of the torso and stimulating the organs and nervous system.

CONTROL THE GATES

The torso consists of three cavities: the thoracic, the abdominal and the pelvic cavities. This is the power chamber of the body. The stronger the power chamber is, the more power you can generate. Just like your biceps or triceps, your power chamber needs to be overloaded to strengthen it. Condensing is like doing a biceps curl for the torso. It is a combination of isometric (condensing while holding) and isotonic (condensing while exhaling) exercises.

To preserve and enhance your inner energy, the gates to each cavity should be regulated. The upper gate is the glottis (throat), the middle gate is the diaphragm, and the lower gate is the pelvic diaphragm. The glottis functions like an air control valve; the diaphragm a piston of an engine; and the pelvic diaphragm is the base of power. When you are able to control the gates of the power chamber, you can harness the amount, intensity, and velocity of force that builds in the body. Steady Breathing is one of the safest methods to practice gate control.

During Steady Breathing, you can practice controlling the gates as follows:

Inhalation: The belly muscles expand and the diaphragm contracts (descends). The glottis opens. The pelvic diaphragm relaxes.

Exhalation: The diaphragm relaxes (ascends). The belly muscles and the pelvic diaphragm begin to contract. The glottis is regulated for controlled exhalation.

Condensing: The diaphragm stops and the glottis closes. The belly muscles and the pelvic diaphragm contract to their maximum.

Release: The diaphragm and the pelvic diaphragm relax. The glottis is regulated. The belly muscles contract.

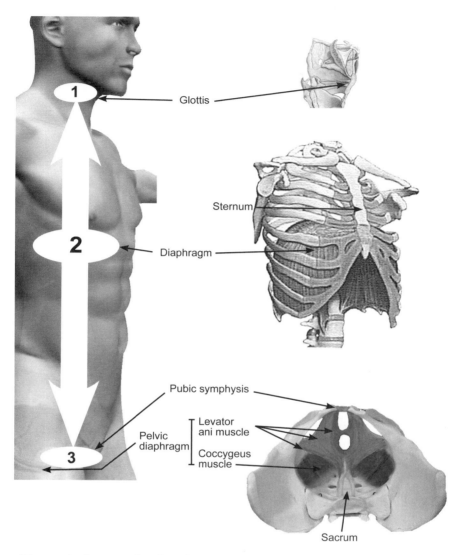

Glottis

Sternum

Diaphragm

Pubic symphysis

Levator
ani muscle

Pelvic
diaphragm

Coccygeus
muscle

Sacrum

The torso is the power chamber of the body. In order to prevent the leakage of condensed energy, the gates of the power chamber, the glottis (1, upper gate) and the pelvic diaphragm (3, lower gate) should be regulated. The diaphragm (2) functions like a piston building the intensity and velocity of the inner force.

Steady Breathing

General Method

1. Stand with your feet shoulder width apart and your hands in front of your lower belly. *Exhale.*

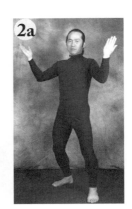

2a-b. Quickly raise your hands in an outward-to-upward circle above your head and *inhale.*

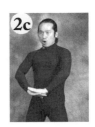

2c. Lower your hands along your median line quickly and *exhale.*

3a-c. Repeat steps 2a to 2c.

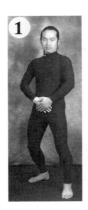

4. Raise your hands above your head and *inhale* to your maximum, then *hold* for 2 seconds.

5. Slowly lower your hands along your median line and begin to *exhale.* Contract the belly muscles progressively and let the diaphragm relax. This is initial condensing.

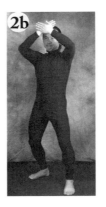

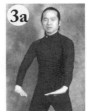

6a-b. At two thirds of exhalation, when your hands arrive in front of your Solar Plexus, abruptly and forcefully contract the muscles of your lower belly and pelvic floor. Begin intense condensing. Continue to lower your hands to the Golden Center for 3-5 seconds while *holding* your breath.

7. When your hands reach your pelvis, snap them outward and force the remaining air out (*exhaling*).

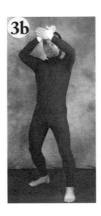

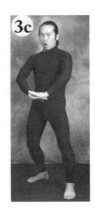

8. Release all of the tension in the body and prepare for the next cycle.

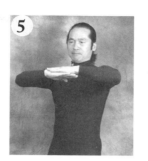

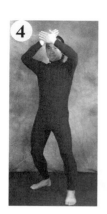

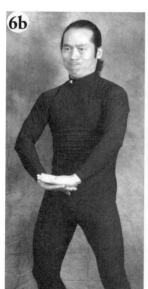

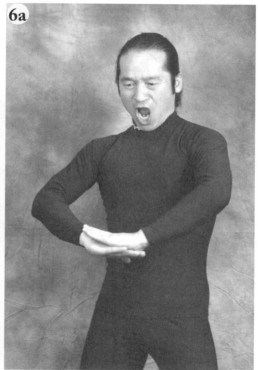

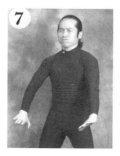

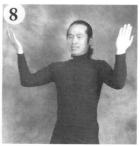

STEADY BREATHING
DETAILED INSTRUCTION

CONDENSING

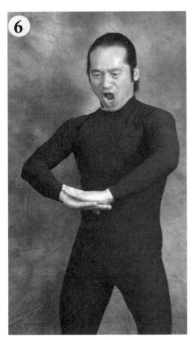

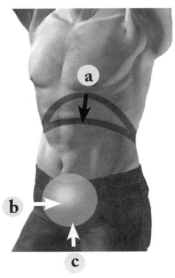

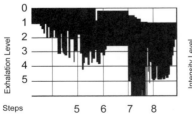

Pause the Diaphragm:

When you hold the breath, keep the diaphragm constant while heightening the contraction of the belly muscles and the pelvic diaphragm. You may adjust the degree of contraction and time based on your feeling.

As your diaphragm descends (a) and your hands arrive in front of your Solar Plexus at the two thirds point of your exhalation, abruptly and forcefully contract the lower belly muscles (b) and increase the inner pressure to maximum (initial condensing). Then, move your hands slowly downward and contract the levator ani muscle on the pelvic floor (c) as if pushing a weight. At the Golden Center, stop your hands, contract all of your inner muscles to maximum and hold your breath for 3-5 seconds before releasing it (intense condensing).

ALTERNATIVE METHOD

Soft Method

1. Stand with your feet shoulder width apart and your hands in front of your lower belly. *Exhale.*

2a. Raise your hands in an out-ward-to-upward circle above your head and *inhale.*

2b-c. Lower your hands along your median line and *exhale.*

3a-c. Repeat steps 2a to 2c.

4. Raise your hands above your head and *inhale* to your maximum, then *hold* for 2 seconds

5. Slowly lower your hands along your median line, gently contracting your belly muscles progressively. *Exhale.*

6. When your hands reach the Golden Center, pause and hold for 3-5 seconds. Gently condense the air while contracting the belly muscles and the pelvic diaphragm.

7. Release the tension and let go.

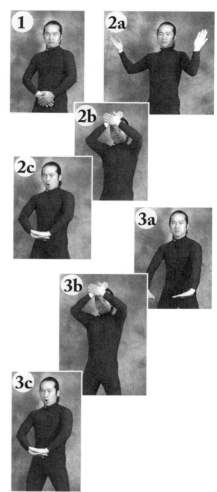

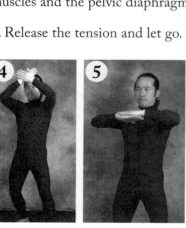

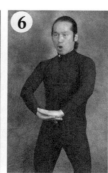

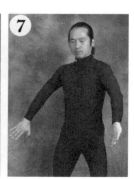

SOUND OF POWER ☯

STEADY BREATHING WITH "*HAA-SSSS-HAA!*"

Exhale forcefully with "Haa" to the 2/3 point while tightening the lower abdomen, and then with abrupt tension tighten the lower abdomen with "Ssss."

1. Expand your belly and take a deep breath through your nose. Exhale through your mouth, making the sound "Haa" while tightening your lower abdomen.
2. Exhale with maximum force at the 2/3-point and make a sound like "Ssss" while clenching your teeth and pulling your tongue back.
3. At 90% of exhalation, further contract the belly muscles and release the tension with the sound "Haa."

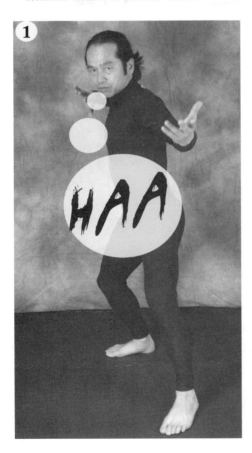

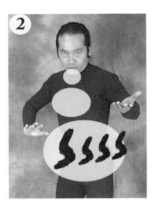

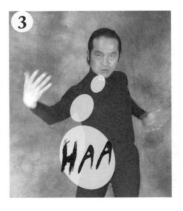

7

STACCATO BREATHING

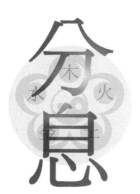

분식

Boon-shik

Strengthen the Inner Gates

Staccato Breathing consists of a long inhalation and short forceful consecutive exhalations. Each exhalation segment is distinctively separate yet rhythmically part of one flowing exhalation.

Staccato Breathing is like brushing the inside of the body to strengthen and massage the eight inner gates: the glottis, trachea, bronchi, Interior Strengthening point, Solar Plexus, umbilicus, Golden Center, and perineum.

You can work on all eight gates or focus on one or several points with each breath. Each time you stop at a particular gate, visualize and feel the inner force at that spot.

Imagine that you are practicing eight short condensing exercises in one breath.

STACCATO BREATHING

General Method

1. Stand with your feet shoulder width apart and your hands in front of your lower belly. *Exhale.*

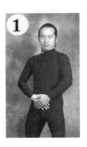
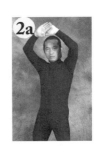

2a. Quickly raise your hands above your head and *inhale.*

2b-c. Circle your hands quickly downward and outward, *exhaling.*

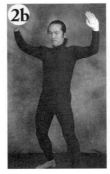
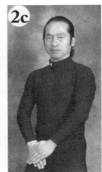

3a-c. Repeat steps 2a to 2c.

4. Raise your hands above your head and *inhale* fully, then *hold* your breath for 2 seconds.

5a. Quickly and forcefully lower your hands to eye level and contract your belly muscles with the first short forceful *exhalation.* Imagine that you are contracting the gate of the throat.

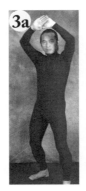
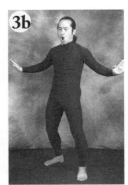

5b-f. Continue to *exhale* and stop at each of the next 5 gates (trachea, bronchi, Solar Plexus, Interior Strengthening point [acupoint CV11], and umbilicus).

6. On the 7th exhalation at the Golden Center, *hold* your breath and hands for 3-5 seconds.

7. While compressing your palms firmly against each other, contract the perineum area.

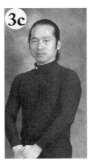
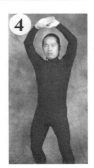

8. Release the tension in your body and let go.

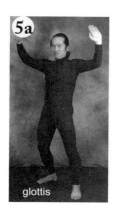

glottis

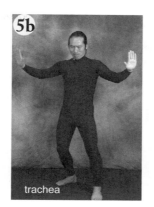

trachea

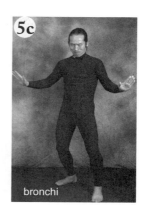

bronchi

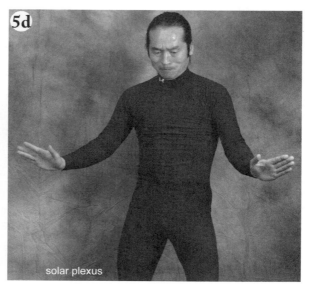

solar plexus

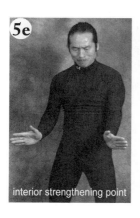

interior strengthening point

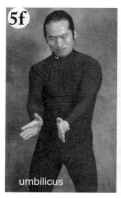

umbilicus

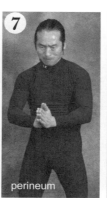

golden center

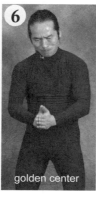

perineum

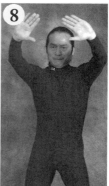

STACCATO BREATHING
DETAILED INSTRUCTION

EIGHT BEAT BREATHING

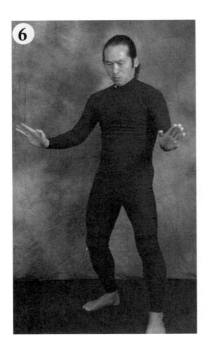

Staccato Breathing is used to strengthen the eight gates of energy passage in the body. The first gate is at the glottis at the top of the neck, the second is the trachea at the entrance to the chest, the third is the bronchi in the lungs, the fourth is the Solar Plexus which is a key nerve network in the mid torso, the fifth is the Interior Strengthening point (acupoint CV11), the sixth is the umbilicus, the seventh is the Golden Center, and the eighth is the perineum in the pelvic floor. The diaphragm stops in synchronization with the focus on each of the eight positions. When you can control the eight gates, you control the source of power in your body.

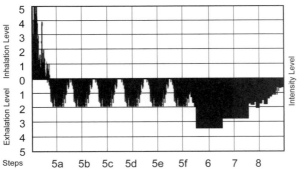

Staccato intensity level:
Prior to the Golden Center breath (steps 5a - 5f), the force level of Staccato Breathing is even. However, you may vary the intensity according to your priorities. If you want to work on the lungs, make the 3rd exhalation (5c) longer and more forceful. The intensity is highest at the Golden Center Condensing stage (6).

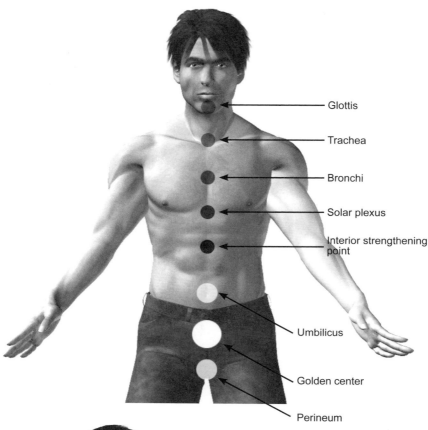

Glottis

Trachea

Bronchi

Solar plexus

Interior strengthening point

Umbilicus

Golden center

Perineum

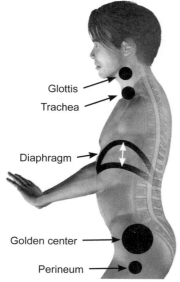

Glottis

Trachea

Diaphragm

Golden center

Perineum

When you practice eight beat breathing (short bursts of exhalation), the prime controllers are the diaphragm and your imagination. As you stop your breath at each of the eight focus points, the diaphragm also stops eight times. That is, the diaphragm makes eight short contractions just as you would do eight repetitions of a biceps curl to strengthen your arm. The initial two gates (glottis and trachea) and the final two gates (Golden Center and perineum) are critical to sealing the body tightly while condensing the air.

ALTERNATIVE METHOD

Soft Method

1. Stand with your feet shoulder width apart and your hands in front of your lower belly. *Exhale.*

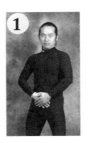
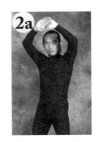

2a. Raise your hands above your head and *inhale.*

2b-c. Circle your hands downward and outward, *exhaling.*

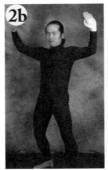
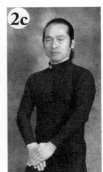

3a-c. Repeat steps 2a to 2c.

4. Raise your hands above your head and *inhale*, then hold your breath for 2 seconds.

5a. Gently lower your hands to eye level and *exhale* a short breath. Imagine gently contracting the throat.

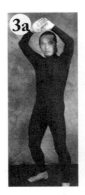
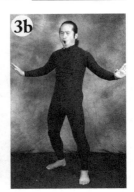

5b-f. Continue to *exhale* and stop at each gate (trachea, bronchi, Solar Plexus, Interior Strengthening point and umbilicus) with short and even exhalations.

6. On the 7th *exhalation* at the Golden Center, hold your breath and hands for 3-5 seconds.

7. While compressing your hands firmly, contract the perineum area.

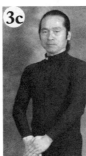
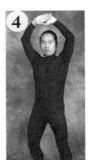

8. Release the tension in your body and let go.

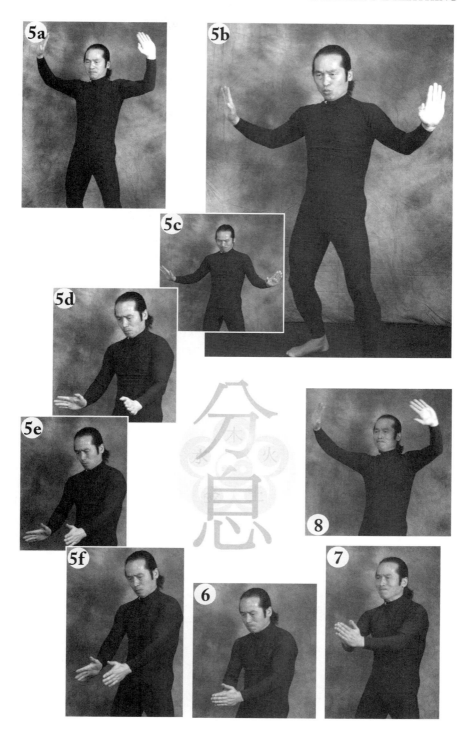

ALTERNATIVE METHOD

Dynamic Method

1. Stand with your feet shoulder width apart and your hands in front of your lower belly. *Exhale.*

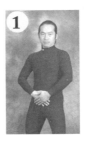
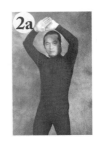

2a. Quickly raise your hands above your head and *inhale*.

2b-c. Circle your hands quickly downward and outward, *exhaling*.

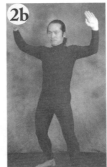
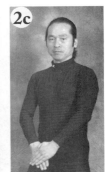

3a-c. Repeat steps 2a to 2c. Move your feet and body around freely, rhythmically stepping forward, backward and sideways in sync with your breathing.

4. Raise your hands above your head and *inhale* to your maximum, then *hold* your breath for 2 seconds.

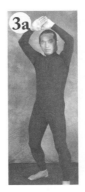
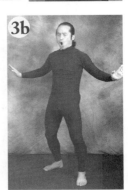

5a-f. Forcefully and quickly lower your hands, stopping at each point of the first six gates, <u>while mobilizing your entire body</u> for maximum muscular contraction.

6. Continue moving around freely as you exhale. On the 7th *exhalation* at the Golden Center, condense the inner force to maximum while holding your breath.

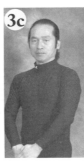
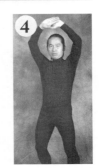

7. Contract the perineum area for 3 seconds.

8. Release the tension in your body and let go.

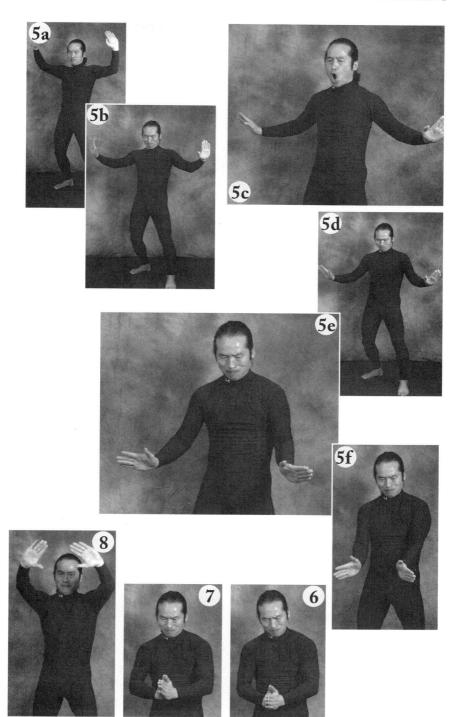

8

HEALING BREATHING

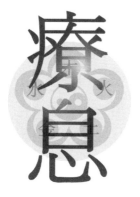

요식

Yo-shik

Restore Optimal Condition

Healing means restoring the body to optimal condition, physically, mentally or spiritually.

Healing Breathing is a natural way of providing abundant oxygen to the body, which nourishes the cells and promotes healthy function of the body at the most basic levels. It raises circulation, detoxifies the body, and stretches and tones the muscles. Taking time to give attention to problem areas and focus on supplying positive energy to your body directly benefits your conscious being.

Review each of the following exercises and select the ones that are applicable to your physical and mental condition at each practice session. You may find that you like to do the full set or that you prefer just a few of the exercises. It's entirely up to you and how you feel on a given day.

Before Beginning Healing Breathing:

There are 10 Healing Breathing exercises. Each exercise stimulates specific areas of the body while applying the principles of Power Breathing.

Each movement has particular points of focus yet you should also maintain your attention to abdominal control.

Most Healing Breathing exercises can also be done using the steady, staccato or explosive breathing methods that you have already learned. Once you feel comfortable with an exercise, experiment with different breathing methods and exercises to increase the intensity and keep your breathing practice fresh.

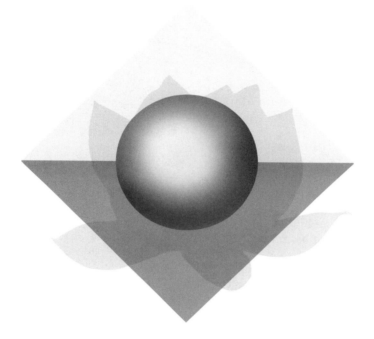

SUPINE POSITION
FILLING THE POND

Water flows to a lower place. Air circulates to a lower density area. Similarly, when you lie on your back, the bones and muscles of your body relax, freed from the stresses of maintaining the structure of the body. The organs rest in newly found space as the forces of gravity pull them toward the spine rather than toward the feet. Fluids are redistributed in the cavities of the torso. This is a moment of rest rather than labor for the body, a time to let your energy flow into the pond of the Golden Center.

COMPRESSION BREATHING

General Method

Purpose: To strengthen the five core muscle groups for breathing

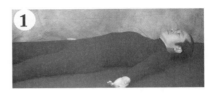

1. Lie back on the floor. Relax for a moment. *Exhale* and *inhale* 3 times.

2. Sink your lower back to the floor and feel the tension in your belly. *Exhale* and *inhale* 3 times.

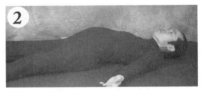

3. Place your palms on your belly. Press your lower back flat on the floor. Expand your belly and chest and *inhale*. As your diaphragm contracts, simultaneously contract your pelvic diaphragm toward the descending diaphragm.

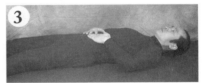

4. *Hold* your breath for 3 seconds.

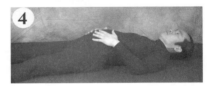

5. Slowly *exhale* and press your belly with your palms. Try to resist the pressure of your palms with the belly muscles (rectus abdominis and transversus abdominis muscles). Relax the diaphragm and pelvic diaphragm progressively while contracting the belly and chest muscles.

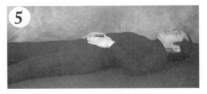

6. At the completion of *exhalation,* you may begin again or rest while doing gentle breathing until you are ready for the next cycle of Compression Breathing.

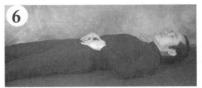

KEY POINT ◉

Five Core Muscle Groups for Power Breathing.

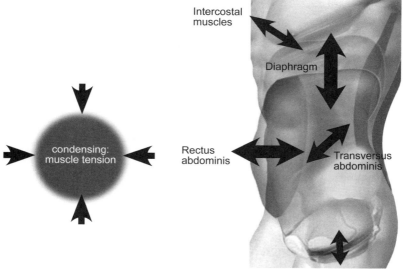

The Core Muscle Groups for Power Breathing

The development of inner or core muscles is something that is rarely addressed in the average fitness program. Many fitness programs and sports focus on the muscles we can see - the arms, shoulders, legs or buttocks. However the core muscles of the torso are just as important to peak performance, in sports and in life. These are the muscles that support the organs, that assist in breathing, that stabilize the spine and pelvis and that assist in gross motor movements like bending, sitting, lifting, and twisting. Powerful movements originate from the center of the body. Before you can move your arms or legs quickly and power-fully, your torso has to be strong and stable. Power Breathing focuses on developing the deep core muscles of the torso to enhance the ability of the torso to transmit power to the arms and legs.

Additionally, the pelvic diaphragm plays a large part in the health and normal function of the reproductive (primarily in women) and urinary organs. Strengthening the pelvic diaphragm, particularly in mid- and late-life, can enhance the health of this important area of the body and prevent health problems like incontinence and pelvic organ prolapse.

COMPRESSION BREATHING

Softer Method

Try this method if you find regular Compression Breathing too intense.

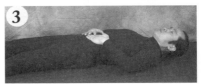

1. Lie back on the floor. Relax for a moment. *Exhale* and *inhale* 3 times.

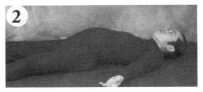

2. Press your lower back to the floor. *Exhale* and *inhale* 3 times.

3. Press your belly with your hands and *inhale*.

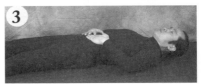

4. *Hold* your breath for 3 seconds.

5. Slowly *exhale* and gently contract the pelvic diaphragm and the belly muscles simultaneously.

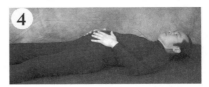

6. At the completion of *exhalation,* you may begin again or rest while doing gentle breathing until you are ready for the next cycle of Compression Breathing.

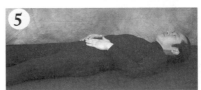

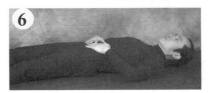

COMPRESSION BREATHING
DETAILED INSTRUCTION

RESTING

Muscles are at rest.

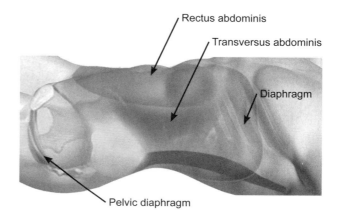

Rectus abdominis

Transversus abdominis

Diaphragm

Pelvic diaphragm

INHALATION

Expand the rectus abdominis and transversus abdominis.

Contract the diaphragm and pelvic diaphragm.

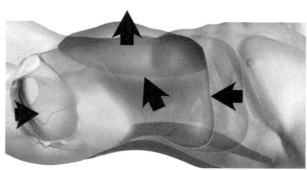

EXHALATION

Contract the rectus abdominis and transversus abdominis.

Relax the diaphragm and pelvic diaphragm.

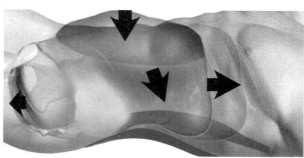

UPLIFTING

General Method

Purpose: To awaken and strengthen the inner muscles of the abdomino-pelvic regions.

1. Lie back on the floor. Relax for a moment. *Exhale* and *inhale* 3 times.

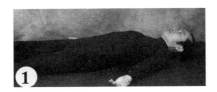

2. Press your lower back to the floor and feel the tension in your belly. *Exhale* and *inhale* 3 times.

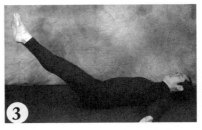

3. *Exhale* slightly and lift your feet 1 to 2 feet above the ground. *Hold* for 3 seconds.

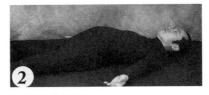

4. Lift your feet to vertical while *inhaling. Hold* for 3 seconds.

5. Slowly lower the feet while fully *exhaling.*

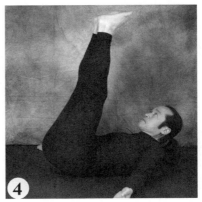

TIPS FOR BEGINNERS:

Lifting the legs while exhaling is harder than doing it while inhaling. It feels like your legs are heavier and your belly muscles work extra-hard. If exhaling is too difficult, try lifting your legs while inhaling at first.

CAUTION:

This exercise may strain your lower back. If you have back pain or a pre-existing back injury, do not perform this exercise.

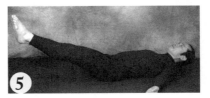

UPLIFTING
DETAILED INSTRUCTION

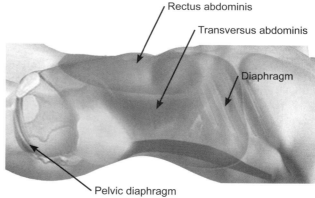

Rectus abdominis

Transversus abdominis

Diaphragm

Pelvic diaphragm

RESTING

Muscles are at rest.

INHALATION

Expand the rectus abdominis and transversus abdominis.

Contract the diaphragm.

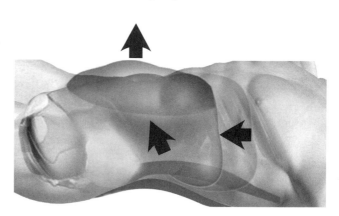

EXHALATION

Contract the rectus abdominis and transversus abdominis.

Also contract the pelvic diaphragm progressively stronger each time you lift the legs.

Relax the diaphragm.

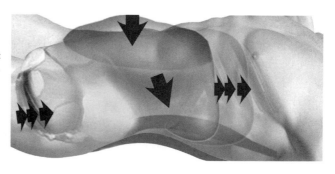

VERTICAL LIFTING

General Method

Purpose: To strengthen the muscles of the upper abdomen and the neck.

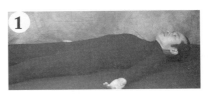

1. Lie back on the floor. Relax for a moment. *Exhale* and *inhale* 3 times.

2. Press your lower back to the floor and feel the tension in your belly. *Exhale* and *inhale*.

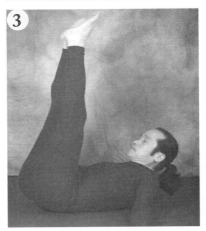

3. *Exhale* and quickly lift your legs to vertical while raising your head and shoulders toward your knees. *Hold* for 3 seconds.

4. At the vertical holding position, *inhale* and *hold* for 3 seconds.

5. Slowly lower your feet and shoulders while *exhaling*.

TRAINING TIPS:

When you initially lift your legs, your lower stomach tenses. When you inhale at the peak of lifting your legs, your torso will expand, like a balloon. Lift your body as much as possible from the floor by raising your head, shoulders and hips. While you hold your breath here, your torso should be bearing a great deal of stress. This is a great way to strengthen your abs.

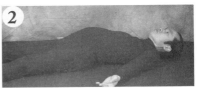

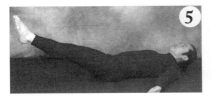

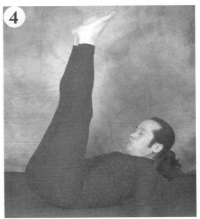

VERTICAL LIFTING
DETAILED INSTRUCTION

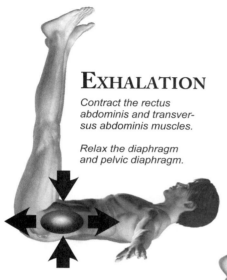

EXHALATION

Contract the rectus abdominis and transversus abdominis muscles.

Relax the diaphragm and pelvic diaphragm.

During exhalation your torso stays flat on the ground while focusing your attention on your lower belly and the weight of your legs.

During inhalation your entire body sits on your lower back muscles, as your hips and head are raised.

POWER TIPS:

For more advanced power practice, breathe in and out 3 to 10 times at position 4. If you are an accomplished athlete, you can inhale and exhale as many as 100 times at this position, to improve your inner power and ab strength. (This method is not recommended for beginners or those who have high blood pressure.)

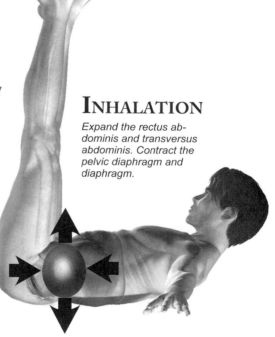

INHALATION

Expand the rectus abdominis and transversus abdominis. Contract the pelvic diaphragm and diaphragm.

CAUTION:

Begin with just a few reps if you don't have strong abs. If you have back or neck pain or a pre-existing injury, do not perform this exercise.

Diamond Pull

General Method

Purpose: To strengthen the muscles of the abdomen.

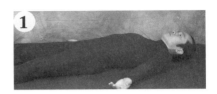

1. Lie back on the floor. Relax for a moment. *Exhale* and *inhale* 3 times.

2. Press your lower back to the floor and feel the tension in your belly. *Exhale* and *inhale*.

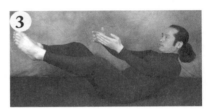

3. Lift your feet and bring them to your chest as you *exhale*.

4. Insert your hands under the calves and hook your ankles with your palm heels. Continue to *exhale*.

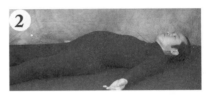

5. Pull your ankles firmly and *inhale* fully. Expand the rectus abdominis and transversus abdominis muscles. Contract the diaphragm and pelvic diaphragm. *Hold* for 3 to 10 seconds.

6. Slowly lower your feet while *exhaling*.

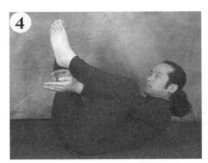

Training Tips:

Advanced practitioners can do up to 20 repetitions without dropping the feet to the ground.

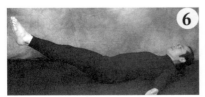

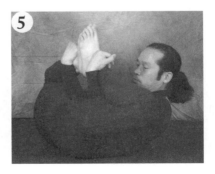

DIAMOND PULL
DETAILED INSTRUCTION

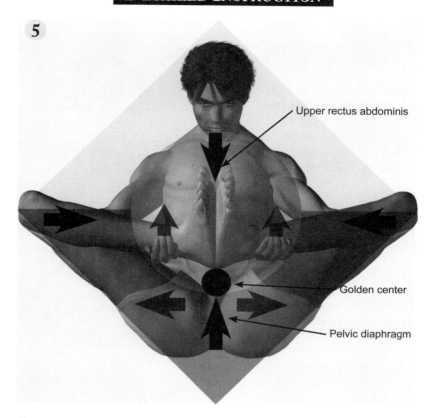

5

Upper rectus abdominis

Golden center

Pelvic diaphragm

INHALATION

Expand the rectus abdominis and transversus abdominis muscles.

Contract the diaphragm and the pelvic diaphragm. The pelvic diaphragm is stretched outward simultaneously by the pulling force of your hips (above).

* All of the energy is flowing toward the Golden Center.

* The contraction of the diaphragm and the pelvic diaphragm condenses the inner pressure in the abdomino-pelvic cavity (right).

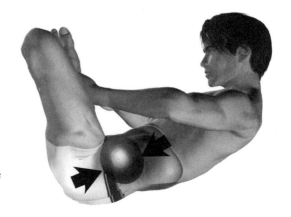

HIP LIFTING 1

General Method

Purpose: To stretch and strengthen the pelvis, groin and chest areas.

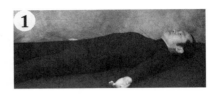

1. Lie back on the floor. Relax for a moment. *Exhale* and *inhale*.

2. Press your lower back to the floor and feel the tension in your belly. *Exhale, inhale* and *exhale*.

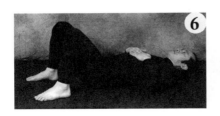

3. Bring your feet close to your buttocks and place your palms on your chest with your fingers interlaced. *Inhale* deeply.

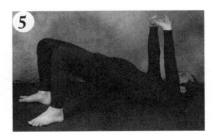

4. Lift your hips and stretch your arms upward with your fingers interlaced (turning your palms to face upward). *Exhale* and *hold* for 3-10 seconds.

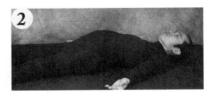

5. *Inhale* deeply, expanding your belly muscles and contracting your diaphragm and pelvic diaphragm. *Hold* for 3-5 seconds.

6. Slowly lower your hips and hands while *exhaling*.

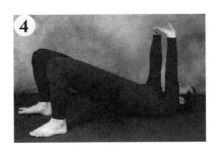

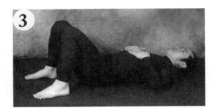

HIP LIFTING 1
DETAILED INSTRUCTION

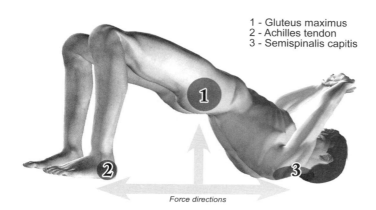

1 - Gluteus maximus
2 - Achilles tendon
3 - Semispinalis capitis

Force directions

LIFT THE HIP AND . .

Stretch the pelvis and the sternum (front of the upper body).

Contract the gluteus maximus (buttocks), press the Achilles tendon to the floor and stretch the semispinalis capitis muscle (rear neck).

INHALE AND . . .

Expand the rectus abdominis and transversus abdominis muscles.

Contract the diaphragm and the pelvic diaphragm.

EXHALE AND . . .

Contract the rectus abdominis and transversus abdominis muscles.

Relax the diaphragm and the pelvic diaphragm.

HIP LIFTING 2

General Method

Purpose: To stretch and strengthen the pelvis, hip and chest areas.

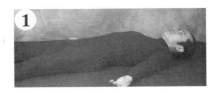

1. Lie back on the floor. Relax for a moment. *Exhale* and *inhale*.

2. Press your lower back to the floor and feel the tension in your belly. *Exhale, inhale* and *exhale*.

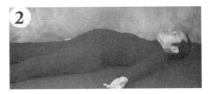

3. Pronate (open) your feet and place your palms on your chest with the fingers interlaced and palms down. *Inhale* deeply.

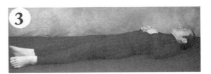

4. Lift your hips and stretch your arms upward, turning your palms upward. *Exhale* and *hold* for 3-10 seconds.

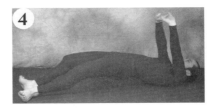

5. *Inhale* deeply while expanding your belly muscles and contracting the diaphragm and pelvic diaphragm. *Hold* 3-5 seconds.

6. Slowly lower your hip and hands while *exhaling*.

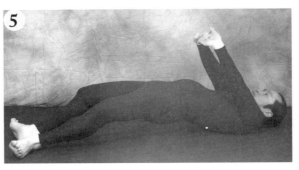

CAUTION:

If you have back problems or a pre-existing back injury, do not perform this exercise.

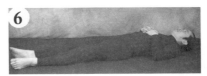

HIP LIFTING 2

DETAILED INSTRUCTION

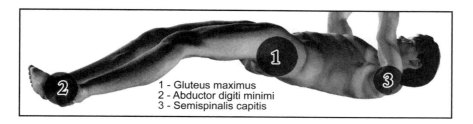

1 - Gluteus maximus
2 - Abductor digiti minimi
3 - Semispinalis capitis

LIFT THE HIPS AND . . .

Stretch the pelvis and the sternum (front of the torso).

Contract the gluteus maximus (1) and stretch the semispinalis capitis muscle in the neck (3).

The upper shoulders and feet (2) support the body's weight.

Energy is directed to the Golden Center.

INHALE AND . . .

Expand the rectus abdominis and transversus abdominis muscles.

Contract the diaphragm and the pelvic diaphragm.

EXHALE AND . . .

Contract the rectus abdominis and transversus abdominis muscles.

Relax the diaphragm and the pelvic diaphragm.

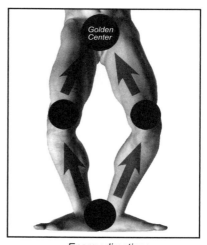

Energy directions

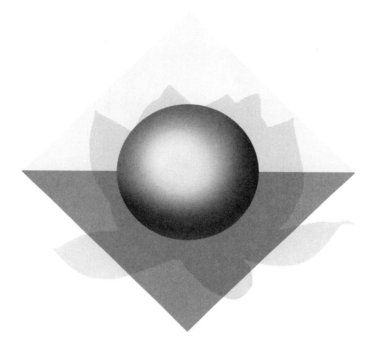

KNEELING POSITION
WATERING THE GARDEN

In the supine position exercises, we worked on *Filling The Pond*. The kneeling position is for *Watering The Garden*. The inner garden of the body is along the spine. Just as water flows into a pond, and once abundant, streams downward, the energy in the body, once filled, rises and circulates. By lowering the organs in the kneeling position, the energy in the body ascends as water descends. By calming the body, the organs rest. As they rest, they reinvigorate themselves. When the garden is enriched, the house becomes lively.

ROLLING CAT

General Method

Purpose: To strengthen the lower abdomen and pelvis with minimal strain. When kneeling, the abdomen can relax and "hang" down. In this position, your abdomen can naturally expand in a very relaxed way.

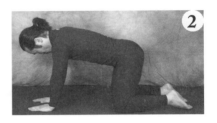

1. Kneel and lower your head in a bowing position. *Exhale.*

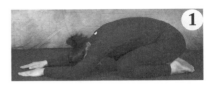

2. Roll forward onto your hands and knees and *inhale* deeply. *Hold* for 3-5 seconds.

3. Raise your head and hips and lower your abdomen while *exhaling.* When your abdomen is fully lowered, *hold* for 3-5 seconds.

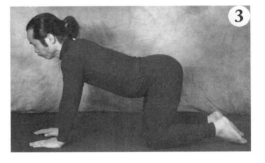

4. *Inhale* while returning to Position 2. *Hold* for 3-5 seconds.

5. Slowly return to the starting position while *exhaling.*

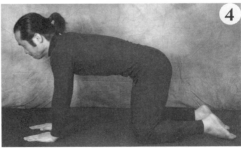

TRAINING TIPS:

When kneeling, it is easy to maintain the natural curves of the spine. Move your hips and middle torso up and down to find the best spinal curve for optimal breathing. Try dropping your shoulders and neck to see what you discover about your posture. You may be able to reinvent this exercise in a way that suits you better.

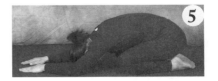

ROLLING CAT
DETAILED INSTRUCTION

3

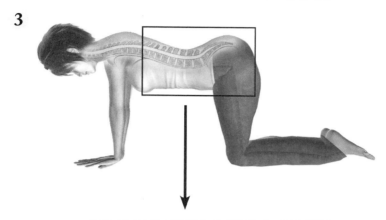

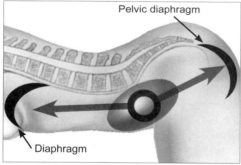

PELVIC STRENGTH TRAINING

The best way to build strength is to increase resistance to muscular contraction. In the Rolling Cat exercise, when the belly is expanded, tense the Core Muscle Groups (rectus abdominis, transversus abdominis, intercostals, diaphragm and pelvic diaphragm). As you exhale and the diaphragm begins to ascend, don't let it go. Contract the pelvic diaphragm like restraining a pulling horse, and pull the diaphragm back slowly and evenly like a tug of war.

INHALATION . . .

Expand the rectus abdominis and transversus abdominis.

Contract the diaphragm and the pelvic diaphragm.

Create maximum tension in the abdominopelvic cavity.

EXHALE AND PELVIC PULL . . .

Contract the rectus abdominis and transversus abdominis.

Contract the pelvic diaphragm and restrain the ascending diaphragm.

ARCHING CAT

General Method

Purpose: To give a deep massage to the abdominopelvic organs. During inhalation, drop your belly as low as possible. During exhalation, raise the center of the torso to the highest possible point.

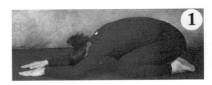

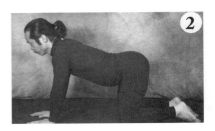

1. Kneel and lower your head in a bowing position. *Exhale.*

2. Roll forward onto your hands and knees and *inhale* deeply. *Hold* for 3 seconds.

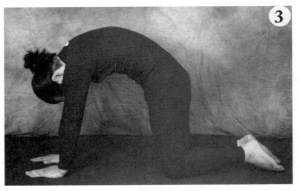

3. Arch upward while exhaling and pulling your belly muscles deeply inward, toward the spine. *Hold* for 3-5 seconds.

4. Return to Position 2 and *inhale.* *Hold* for 3 seconds.

5. Slowly return to Position 1 while *exhaling.*

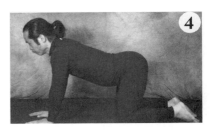

T`RAINING` T`IPS`:

Always let your body guide you. Only push your limits based on how much you have progressed. If you have any unusual or prolonged discomfort, stop and take a break or move on to a different exercise.

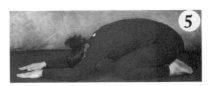

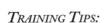

ARCHING CAT
DETAILED INSTRUCTION

3

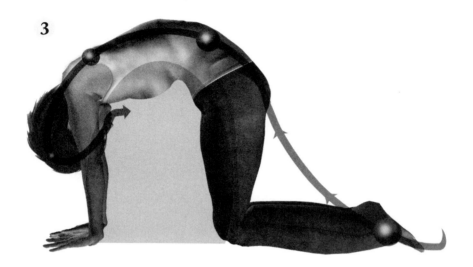

HOUSE CLEANING

Toxins and excess carbon dioxide in the body burden the system. Through Power Breathing, you can increase circulation and cleanse your body. When you are tired, 10 repetitions of Arching Cat can leave you feeling refreshed and revitalized. When you arch and exhale, imagine that you have a long tail and begin to exhale from the end of it. As you arch, pull your belly muscles in and upward to put pressure on your abdominal and chest cavities and expel all of the air from your body.

INHALATION

Expand the rectus abdominis and transversus abdominis. Drop your belly downward.

Contract the diaphragm and relax the pelvic diaphragm.

EXHALE FROM THE TAIL

Arch your back progressively to the highest point while contracting the rectus abdominis and transversus abdominis muscles.

As you exhale, imagine exhaling from the tip of your tail, through your torso, chest, neck and head. Suck your belly muscles upward and inward to press the air out fully.

PELVIS OPENING

General Method

Purpose: To release tension in the pelvis.

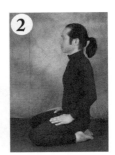
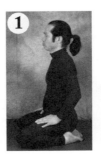

1. Kneel and *inhale* deeply.

2. *Exhale* deeply. Contract the diaphragm and the belly muscles slowly and deeply to expel all of the air, pushing upward from the pelvic floor.

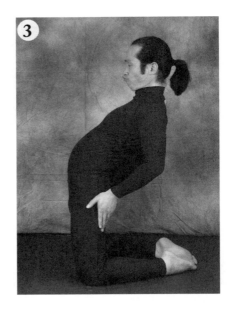

3. Lift your hips, push your pelvis forward and *inhale* deeply. As you condense the air to the lower belly, relax and drop your shoulders. Contract the diaphragm muscles and at maximum tension, *hold* for 3-10 seconds.

4. *Exhale* slowly and return your hips to below your torso. At this time squeeze your knees inward and contract the pelvic floor muscles. Do everything slowly and steadily.

5. As you sit back, gently contract your lower belly muscles and pelvic diaphragm and complete a full *exhalation.*

TRAINING TIPS:

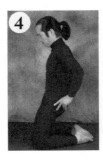

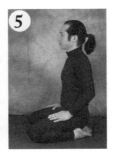

This exercise is harder than it looks. If you are short of breath, go easy, reducing the length of the breath. As you improve, do each segment as slowly as possible. Remember, there is not only one way of doing each exercise. Be creative!

PELVIS OPENING
DETAILED INSTRUCTION

3

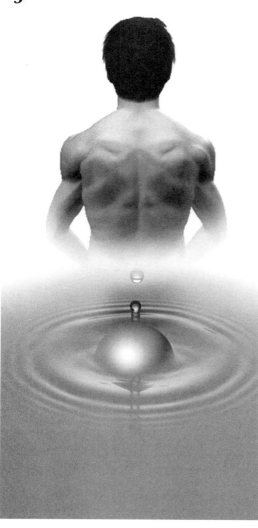

DROPPING THE SHOULDERS

Drop your shoulders as if they are pulled by an inner weight. The shoulders should not have any tension in them; they should stay passive, like a rock sinking in a pond.

INHALATION

Expand the rectus abdominis and transversus abdominis muscles. Arch your body slightly backward.

Contract the diaphragm and relax the pelvic diaphragm.

EXHALE AND TENSE THE PELVIS

Lean your torso slightly forward. Slowly contract the rectus abdominis and transversus abdominis. Squeeze the thighs inward and tense the pelvis.

As you sit, expel the last drop of the air by contracting the lower belly muscles and the pelvic diaphragm.

CAMEL POSITION

General Method

Purpose: To stretch the thoracic, abdominal and pelvic cavities.

1. Kneel with your knees open.

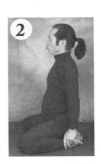

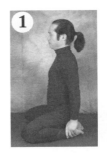

2. *Inhale* deeply. Drop your shoulders. Contract the diaphragm and pelvic diaphragm and condense the air downward.

3. Lift your hips and push your pelvis forward. Relax the pelvic diaphragm and arch your body backward. *Exhale. Hold* for 3-5 seconds and try to relax.

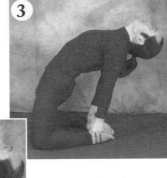

4. *Inhale* deeply, expanding your belly. When the belly becomes full, condense it by contracting the diaphragm and pelvic diaphragm. *Hold* for 3-5 seconds. Then relax the pelvic diaphragm and slide the condensed air ball down toward the pelvis.

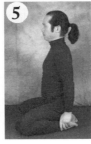

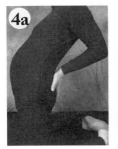

5. *Exhale* and return to Position 1.

<u>*CAUTION:*</u>

If you have back pain, do not attempt this exercise. To make the exercise easier, support your lower back with your hands (4A) rather than holding your ankles.

CAMEL POSITION
DETAILED INSTRUCTION

4

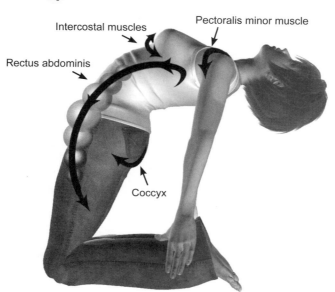

Intercostal muscles

Pectoralis minor muscle

Rectus abdominis

Coccyx

SINKING THE GOLDEN BALL

In this arched Camel Position you are pushing the pelvis forward and contracting (tucking) the coccyx area while stretching the pectoralis minor muscle in the upper chest and the intercostal muscles. As you push the torso further forward, you can feel the rectus abdominis stretching. Just let it go and expand the belly. With your active imagination and muscular control push the condensed ball of energy from the Solar Plexus down to the umbilicus, the Golden Center and beyond, then let it sink wherever it might go. When you return to kneeling, exhale slowly.

INHALATION

Expand the rectus abdominis and transversus abdominis muscles as you arch your body backward.

Contract the diaphragm and coccyx area (buttocks). Relax the pelvic diaphragm.

EXHALE

Lean your torso slightly forward. Slowly contract the rectus abdominis and transversus abdominis.

As you sit, expel the last drop of the air by contracting the lower belly muscles and the pelvic diaphragm.

FROG POSITION

General Method

Purpose: To relax and stretch the pelvic muscles.

1. Kneel with your knees open. *Inhale* and *exhale.*

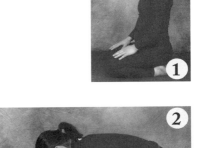

2. Glide your hands forward and move onto your knees and elbows. *Inhale. Hold* for 3 seconds.

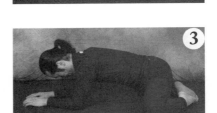

3. *Exhale* and open your knees as wide as possible. Relax your pelvis. *Hold* for 3-10 seconds.

4. *Inhale* and lower your belly to the floor, continuing to relax your pelvis.

5. *Exhale* and bring back your knees together.

6. Return to kneeling and prepare for the next cycle.

TRAINING TIPS:
During Step 4 inhalation, sink your whole body like your belly is filled with lead.

CAUTION:
Be sure to stretch the pelvis thoroughly before attempting a full pelvis opening in Step 4.

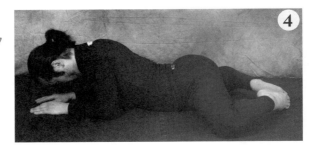

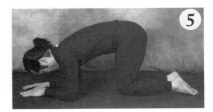

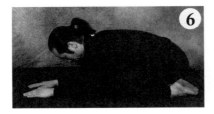

FROG POSITION
DETAILED INSTRUCTION

4

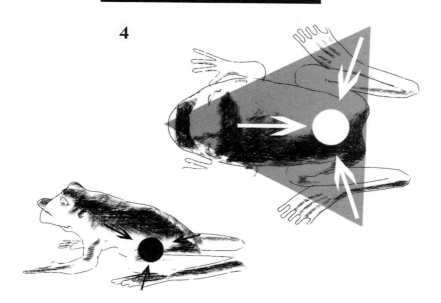

FROG AT REST

The posture of the limbs and trunk at rest is important for well-being. This resting frog position is symmetrical and balanced with the center of the gravity low on the ground, where the trunk is able to rest.

Relax the pelvis, rest your hands and let your body sink toward the Golden Center. Feel the power of the condensed energy spreading across your body.

Deeply inhale and exhale. Feel the stretching inner muscles and building forces in the cavities filling your body like a balloon of fresh oxygen. Push out all of the toxins and energize the cells.

INHALATION

Expand the rectus abdominis and transversus abdominis. Lower your belly as far as possible. You may move your body slightly forward for easier breathing.

Contract the diaphragm and coccyx area. Relax the pelvic diaphragm.

EXHALE

Slowly contract the rectus abdominis and transversus abdominis muscles and the pelvic diaphragm.

As you expel the last drop of air, move your body slightly to the rear for a complete exhalation.

COOL DOWN

General Method

Purpose: To relax and prepare to return to daily activities.

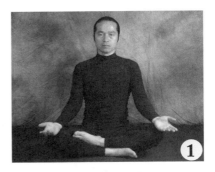

1. Sit with your legs crossed. Align your head, neck and spine vertically. Drop your shoulders and relax your arms.

2. Put your right hand on top of your top ankle with your palms facing upward. Rest your left hand on top of your right palm with your palm facing upward. Keep your mouth closed loosely, teeth slightly apart and tongue relaxed. Close your eyes gently.

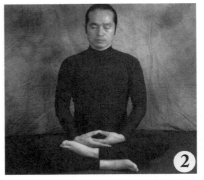

3. *Exhale* slowly and evenly, and then *inhale* through your nose.

Repeat 5-10 times.

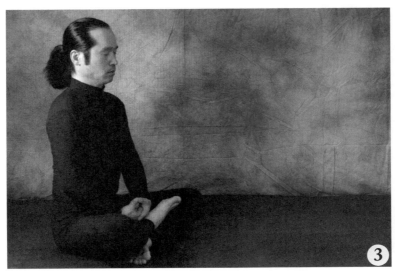

9

POWER BREATHING WORKOUTS

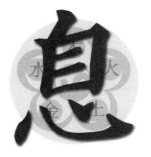

Breathing

Now that you have learned and practiced the individual Power Breathing exercises, you are ready to put the exercises together in workouts.

The workouts in this chapter are just a few of the possible ways of combining the exercises of Power Breathing. They vary from short and easy (One Minute Breathing) to challenging (Power Workout). Each has been designed with a particular goal in mind: refreshing the mind, toning the body, strengthening for sports or relieving stress.

Based on these examples, be creative and design your own ideal Power Breathing Workout!

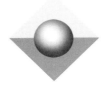 # ONE MINUTE WORKOUT

When you don't have a lot of time, practice One Minute Breathing. It is a short routine but it has all of the elements of Power Breathing. It begins with modified Gentle Breathing then moves on to Explosive, Steady and Staccato Breathing and ends with Cool Down Breathing.

1 Modified Gentle Breathing

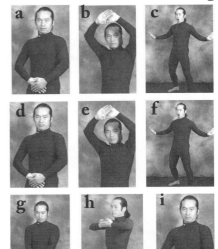

1. Modified Gentle Breathing:

a. *Exhale* from ready position.

b. Raise your arms up and *inhale*.

c-d. Circle your arms outward and *exhale*.

e-f. Repeat b-c.

g. Bring your palms together in front of the Golden Center.

h. Raise your hands to your chest with your palms facing you and *inhale*.

i. Lower your hands to the Golden Center and *exhale*.

2. Explosive Breathing:

a-e. Raise your arms *inhaling* and circle your arms outward *exhaling*.

f-g. *Exhale* and begin initial condensing.

2 Explosive Breathing

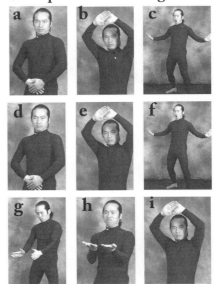

h. Tense your muscles for intense condensing while raising your hands upward.

i. Release.

j. Let go and prepare for Steady Breathing with a deep *exhalation*.

3. Steady Breathing:

a-c. As soon as the hands arrive at the Golden Center, circle out and upward, *inhaling*.

d. Press the hands down along the median line and *exhale*.

e-f. Repeat a-c.

g-h. *Exhale* sharply and condense for 5 seconds until your hands reach the Golden Center.

i. Release with deep *exhalation*.

j-k. Circle your hands upward naturally and *inhale*.

l. Lower your hands along the median line and *exhale*. Get ready for Staccato Breathing.

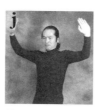

3 Steady Breathing

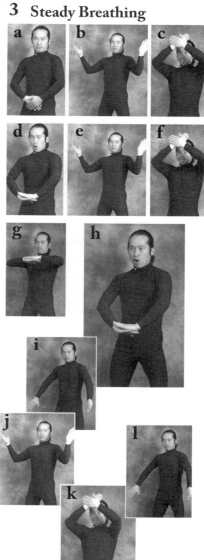

4. Staccato Breathing:

a-d. Raise your arms above your head, *inhaling*, and circle your arms down and outward, *exhaling*.

e. Raise your arms again, *inhaling*.

f. Begin the first condensing (glottis) with a short spurt of *exhalation*.

g-k. Continue to *exhale* and stop at each gate (trachea, bronchi, Solar Plexus, Interior Strengthening point and umbilicus) with short and even *exhalations*.

l. On the 7th *exhalation* at the Golden Center, hold your breath and hands for 3-5 seconds.

m. While compressing your hands firmly, contract the perineum area.

n-o. Release the tension in your body and let go.

4 Staccato Breathing

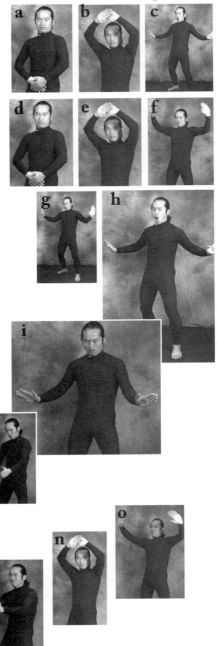

5. Cool Down Breathing:

a. *Exhale* from ready position.

b. Raise your arms up and *inhale*.

c-d. Circle arms outward and *exhale*.

e-f. Repeat b-c.

g. Bring your palms together in front of the Golden Center.

h. Raise your hands to your chest with your palms facing you and *inhale*.

i. Lower your hands to the Golden Center and exhale.

This concludes
One Minute Power Breathing.

Total practice time: 60 seconds

5 Cool Down Breathing

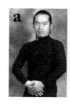
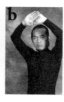

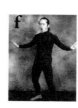
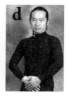
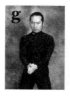
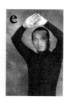
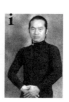

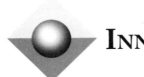 # INNER TUNE-UP

Inner Tune-up stretches the muscles in the torso, arms and hands (Sunrise Breathing), tones the chest muscles and lungs (Awakening Lotus), and strengthens the diaphragm (Diamond Breathing).

Repetitions:

1. Sunrise Breathing: 3 times
2. Awakening Lotus: 3 times
3. Diamond Breathing: 3 times
4. Sunrise Breathing: once
5. Awakening Lotus: once

Approximate Cycle Time:

For Beginners: 15 seconds per breath cycle.

For intermediate: 15-20 seconds per breath cycle.

For advanced: 20-30 seconds per breath cycle.

For expert: 30-45 seconds per breath cycle.

1 Sunrise Breathing

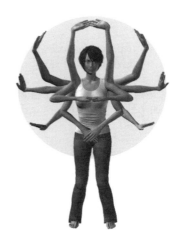

Stretch with Sunrise Breathing. (instruction on page 50)

- Focus on fully stretching your arms and chest muscles.
- Expand your chest vertically.
- Inhale as deeply as you can.
- Hold at the top for greater oxygen intake.
- Slowly exhale and circle your hands downward while fully stretching your arms (keeping your hands bent).
- Be aware of your chest as the center of the exercise.
- Exhale completely.

Repeat 3 times freely.

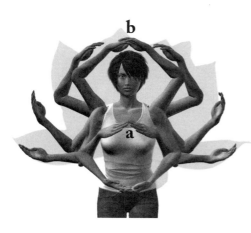

2 Awakening Lotus

Tone your lungs with Awakening Lotus. (instruction on page 52)

- Focus on opening and massaging your lungs through gentle arm circles.
- Awaken your lungs with a small blossoming circle (a).
- Inhale and exhale quietly.
- Expand your lungs with a full blossoming lotus circle (b).
- Inhale deeply, exhale gently.

Repeat 3 times slowly.

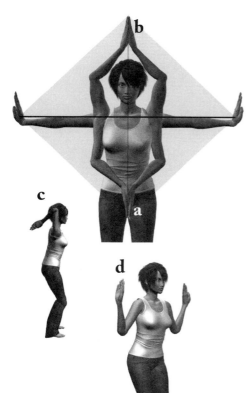

3 Diamond Breathing

Strengthen your diaphragm with Diamond Breathing. (instruction on page 54)

- Focus on controlling your diaphragm.
- Take a long, deep breath (a to b).
- Continue to inhale. Imagine you are expanding the lungs vertically (b to c).
- Lower your elbows to the sides and open your chest. Continue to inhale and imagine you are expanding the lungs horizontally. (c to d).
- Slowly and forcefully exhale.

Repeat 3 times slowly.

* CAUTION: Inhalation of Diamond Breathing is twice as long as exhalation. You may adjust the length of each breathing for your comfort.

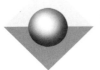 # TEN MINUTE WORKOUT

SAMPLE 1: Power Breathing Trio

Methods: Standing, sitting on chair, sitting on the floor, kneeling

Warm-up:

Sunrise Breathing - 3 reps (page 50)
Awakening Lotus - 3 reps (page 52)
Diamond Breathing - 3 reps (page 54)

Core Exercises:

Explosive Breathing - 4 reps (page 69)
Steady Breathing - 4 reps (page 87)
Staccato Breathing - 4 reps (page 95)

Cool-down:

Cool Down Breathing (page 134)

SAMPLE 2: Floor Exercises

Methods: Explosive Breathing on the floor

Warm-up:

Compression Breathing (page 110)

Core Exercises:

Uplifting - 3 reps (page 112)
Diamond Pull - 3 reps (page 116)
Hip Lifting 1- 3 reps (page 118)
Rolling Cat - 3 reps (page 124)
Arching Cat - 3 reps (page 126)

Cool-down:

Cool Down Breathing (page 134)

TRAINING TIPS:

One cycle of each exercise takes approximately 30 seconds for intermediate and advanced practitioners. If you are a beginner do shorter breathing cycles with more repetitions to bring the total practice time to ten minutes.

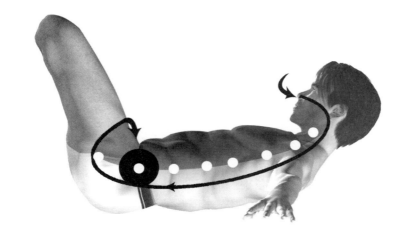

 # DIAMOND PULL

Diamond Pull is an exercise for strengthening the energy channel that runs through the center of the torso. It can be practiced with all three of the Power Breathing methods introduced in this book: explosive, steady and staccato. The Explosive method develops the capacity of the entrance (nostrils, first arrow), the force of the energy flow (second arrow) and the power of the Golden Center (black circle). The Steady method develops the strength of the median muscles to stabilize the central energy path (grey area of the torso). The Staccato method strengthens the eight points of the inner gates (white dots).

By following this example, any of the Healing Breathing exercises can be done with three Power Breathing methods.

1. Explosive Method

Develop the capacity of the airways, the force of the energy flow and inner power (details on page 116).

- While lifting your legs, *exhale* and focus on the flow of the air exiting from the body through your lungs and nostrils.
- 1a. *Inhale.* Focus on the flow of the incoming air to the Golden Center (black circle). Hold for 3-5 seconds.
- At position 1a, *exhale* and *inhale* 5 times.
- After each *inhalation*, hold for 3-5 seconds. Support your entire body on your lower back.

Repeat 3 sets. Each set is 1 minute.

1 Explosive Method

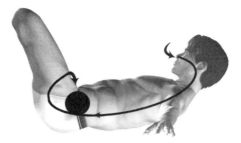

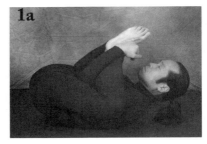

2. Steady Method

Strengthen the median muscles to stabilize the central energy path (details on page 90).

- 2a. Stretch your arms up. *Inhale.*
- 2b. Raise your hands toward your legs and *exhale.* Begin to lift your torso slowly.
- 2c. Continue lifting and *exhale.* Focus on the progressive tension from the neck to the Golden Center.
- 2d. Pull your legs and *inhale.* Hold for 3-5 seconds focusing on the tension in the Golden Center. Return to 2a position. *Exhale.*

Repeat 5 sets. Each set is 30 seconds.

2 Steady Method

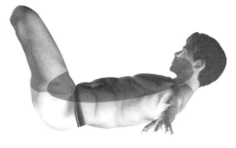

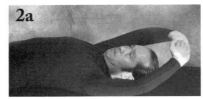

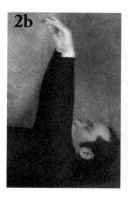

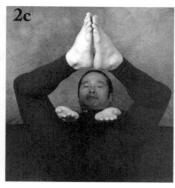

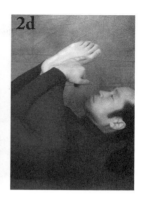

3. Staccato Method

Strengthen the eight points of the inner gates (white dots) (details on page 96).

- 3a. *Inhale.* Begin to open your arms while lifting your torso for Staccato Breathing, *exhaling.*
- With even *exhalations,* progressively lift your body higher and stop at the 6 gates (glottis, trachea, bronchi, Solar Plexus, Interior Strengthening point, and umbilicus).
- 3b. At the 7th gate, the Golden Center, hold for 3-5 seconds.
- 3c. At the 8th gate of the perineum, hold your legs and *exhale* completely.
- *Inhale* and return to 3a.

Repeat 3 sets. Each set in 30 seconds.

TRAINING TIPS:

Be creative in moving your hands, arms and legs. The degree of lifting your body depends on your physical condition. As long as you feel tension at each gate, you are doing fine. If the eight gates are too hard, do a few at first. Be steady in practice!

3 Staccato Method

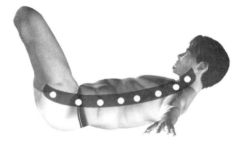

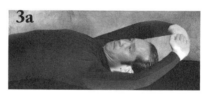

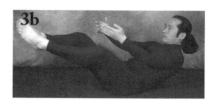

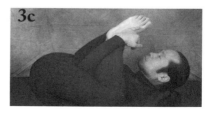

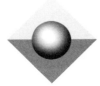 # STRESS RELIEF WORKOUT

Goal: To remove stiffness and tension in your muscles of the back, shoulders and neck, and in turn, to reduce or remove back pain, neck pain, headache, anxiety, and insomnia due to stress.

Level: All levels
Repetition: 5–10 times

1. Sunrise Breathing *(Details on page 50)*

Raise your arms up and stretch the muscles of your arms, shoulders, neck, chest and lower back.

- Stretch out as far as you can.
- *Inhale* as deeply as you can.
- *Exhale* as slowly as you can.

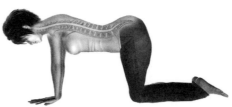

2. Sleeping Turtle *(Details on page 58)*

Expand your torso and stretch the muscles of the entire torso.

- *Inhale* deeply.
- Expand the torso horizontally and vertically, especially the back muscles.
- *Exhale* as slowly as you can.

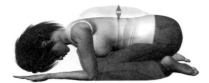

3. Rolling Cat *(Details on page 124)*

Stretch and strengthen the pelvis, groin and chest areas.

- Kneel in bowing position and *exhale*.
- In cat position, *inhale* deeply.
- Arch your torso downward.
- Hold for 3-5 seconds.
- Back to kneeling bow position. *Exhale.*

4. Hip Lifting 1 *(Details on page 118)*

Stretch and strengthen the pelvis and chest muscles.

- Lie back and *exhale.*
- Raise your hips and arms, and *inhale* deeply.
- Hold for 3-5 seconds.
- Lower your hips and arms. *Exhale.*

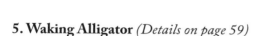

5. Waking Alligator *(Details on page 59)*

Release tension in the pelvic cavity.

- Lie on your stomach and *exhale.*
- Raise your torso gently and *inhale* deeply.
- Hold for 3-5 seconds while pressing the floor with your lower belly.
- Lower your torso. *Exhale.*

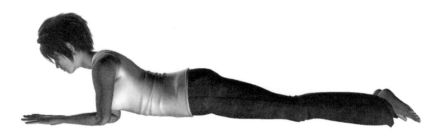

6. End with Sleeping Turtle *(Details on page 58)*

Rest your organs with Gentle Breathing.

- *Inhale* gently.
- Expand the torso and feel the inner pressure.
- *Exhale* slowly and feel the organs hanging down from the tree of the spine.

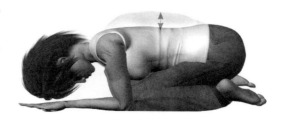

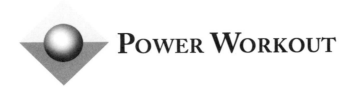

POWER WORKOUT

Goal: To enhance inner power by strengthening the core muscles and breathing capacity.

Level: Strenuous to challenging (not for those who have back pain or injury)

1. Vertical Lifting *(Details on page 114)*

Lift your legs vertically.
Inhale and hold for 3-5 seconds and *exhale*.
Repetitions: 5-20 times.

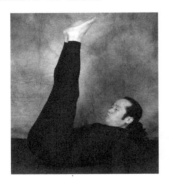

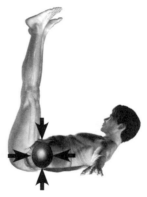

2. Hip Lifting 2 *(Details on page 120)*

Lie back and *Inhale* .
Lift your hips and arms and *exhale*.
Hold for 3-5 seconds.
Lower your body and *inhale*.
Repetitions: 5-20 times.

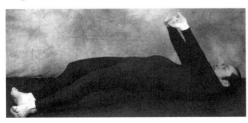

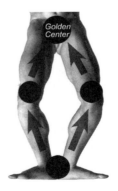

3. Diamond Pull *(Details on page 116)*

Lie back and *inhale.*
Lift your legs and pull. *Exhale.*
Inhale in the position shown below and hold for 3-5 seconds
then *exhale.*
Repetitions: 5-20 times.

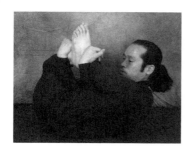 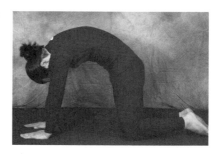

4. Arching Cat *(Details on page 126)*

In a hands and knees position,
lift your torso as high as you can
and *exhale.*
Lower your torso and *inhale.*
Repetitions: 5-10 times.

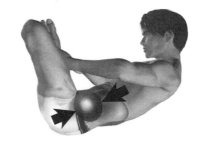

5. Camel Position *(Details on page 130)*

In a kneeling position, bend your torso backward and *inhale* deeply.
Hold for 3-5 seconds.
Back to kneeling position and *inhale.*
Repetitions: 5 times.

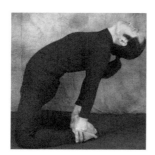 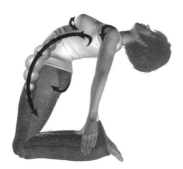

ABOUT THE AUTHOR

Sang H. Kim is the creator of Power Breathing for Life. He is the author of international bestsellers *Ultimate Flexibility, Ultimate Fitness Through Martial Arts,* and *1001 Ways to Motivate Yourself and Others.* His books have been translated into 22 languages. He has been featured or reviewed in Hartford Current, San Francisco Sun Reporter, Inner-self Magazine, The Observer, The New York Times, El Nacional, Dallas Observer, Donga Newspaper-Seoul, Chosun Daily-Seoul, Delta Sky, Fighter's Magazine-UK, Cumbernauld Gazette-Scotland, Memphis Business Journal and hundreds more publications.

An internationally respected authority on health and fitness and martial arts training, Sang H. Kim has taught tens of thousands of students in seminars and workshops in North America, Europe, and Asia. He is a certified 8th degree black belt and martial arts instructor as well as the holder of an MS degree in Sports Science and Ph.D. in Sports Media Studies. As the founder of Power Breathing for Life, he is recognized as one of the most innovative masters of healthy living. He divides his time among Southwest, East coast and Asia, writing and practicing martial arts and Power Breathing.

INDEX

POWER BREATHING DVD IS AVAILABLE!

Revitalize your energy with Power Breathing. Martial arts expert and Power Breathing for Life creator Sang H. Kim guides you through easy to follow breathing exercises that you can do anywhere, in as little as sixty seconds, to relieve stress, increase your fitness level and feel better instantly.

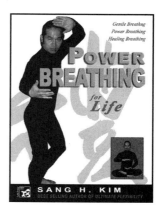

New to breathing exercises? Start with Gentle Breathing, a simple way to reconnect with your body and begin your journey toward renewed energy. When you're ready, the core Power Breathing exercises of Steady, Staccato and Explosive breathing combine to create a total body energizing workout that will leave you feeling refreshed and revitalized. Finally, give attention to problem areas with Healing Breathing – ten exercises to release tension and promote flexibility through controlled breathing.

Sang H. Kim has created this instructional DVD detailing the Power Breathing methods he has use for over 3 decades as part of his daily martial arts training. Power Breathing is an excellent way of improving lung capacity, strengthening the core mucles of the torso, increasing stamina, reducing stress and channeling inner energy. Its principles can be applied to martial arts training, yoga, tai chi and many aerobic sports. The DVD includes both instruction and follow along workouts.

DVD DETAILS:

* Format: Color, DVD-Video, NTSC
* UPC: 823327206722
* Number of discs: 1
* Run Time: 75 minutes

AVAILABLE FROM:
www.TurtlePress.com
www.amazon.com

For more information on Power Breathing, go to:
www.PowerBreathingForLife.com